その症候、英語で言えますか？

はじめに覚える335症候と ついでに覚える1000の関連語

著：近藤真治
英文校閲・ナレーター：Wayne Malcolm
編集協力：飯野 哲

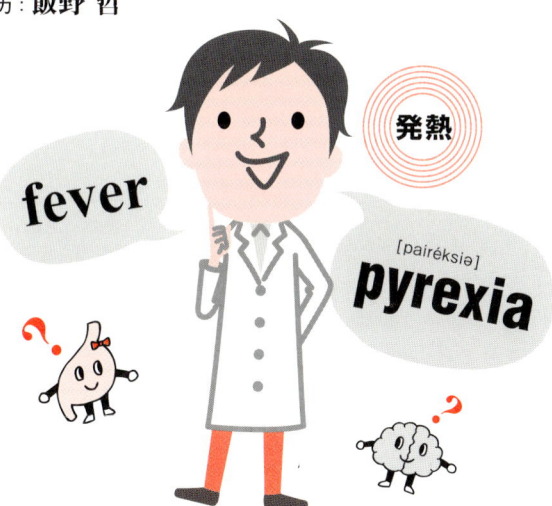

発熱

fever

[pairéksiə]
pyrexia

羊土社

【注意事項】本書の情報について

　本書に記載されている内容は，発行時点における最新の情報に基づき，正確を期するよう，執筆者，監修・編者ならびに出版社はそれぞれ最善の努力を払っております．しかし科学・医学・医療の進歩により，定義や概念，技術の操作方法や診療の方針が変更となり，本書をご使用になる時点においては記載された内容が正確かつ完全ではなくなる場合がございます．また，本書に記載されている企業名や商品名，URL等の情報が予告なく変更される場合もございますのでご了承ください．

はじめに

　医師による診察は，患者の症候を把握することから始まります．正確な診断や適切な治療は，さまざまな症候を正しく理解して初めて可能となります．この意味で，症候に関する知識は，医療のプロとしての医師の最も基本的な能力ということができます．

　医学英語の学習においても事情は変わりません．専門誌や学会，インターネット等を通じて海外のさまざまな症例を学ぶ際，症候に関する用語や表現の理解は必要不可欠といえます．例えば，世界で最も読まれている症例報告とされる *The New England Journal of Medicine* の Case Records に次のような記述があります（症候を下線で表示）．

　There was a systolic ejection murmur at the right upper sternal border. An examination revealed a few beats of horizontal nystagmus and mild ataxia. The Romberg test was positive.

　症候の英語を理解することが英文症例報告を読むうえでの前提となることは，この例からも明らかです．

　症候の英語を学ぶ場合，単に英語を日本語に置き換えるだけでなく，その学術的な意味を理解することが重要となります．上の例にある "ataxia" を「運動失調」と訳すだけでは不十分で，それが随意運動中の筋活動の協調障害を意味し，小脳や脊髄後索の疾患を示唆すること等を理解して初めてその用語を習得したということができます．本書では，335の基本症候の定義が英語と日本語で記述されていますので，各症候の学術的意味のみならず，「随意運動（voluntary movement）」「小脳（cerebellum）」「脊髄（spinal cord）」「後索（posterior funiculus）」等の関連語やそれ

らが使用される文脈も同時に学ぶことができます．本書による学習が終了した暁には，1,300を超える専門用語が身についていることでしょう．なお，本書に掲載した見出し語の発音は，すべて音声データとしてダウンロードが可能です．音声を繰り返し聞き，また自分でも発音してみることで，医学英語独特の発音やアクセントの特徴をつかんでください．

本書の執筆に当たっては，『医師国家試験出題基準』（厚生労働省），『ステッドマン医学大辞典』（メジカルビュー社），『*Stedman's Medical Dictionary*』（LWW），『医学大辞典』（医学書院），『医学英和辞典』（研究社）等を参照しました．基礎レベルの医学英語からのステップアップを考えている幅広い方々に本書を活用していただければ幸いです．

最後になりましたが，本書の英文校閲と見出し語のナレーションを担当していただいた福井大学語学センターのWayne Malcolm先生，解剖図の作成にご協力いただいた福井大学医学部の飯野哲先生，本書の出版に多大なご尽力をいただいた株式会社羊土社編集部の久本容子さんと溝井レナさんに厚く御礼申し上げます．

2014年9月

愛知医科大学看護学部教授
近藤真治

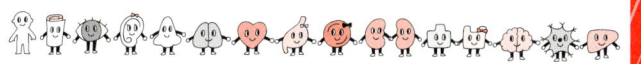

Contents

はじめに

掲載症候(見出し語)一覧 ……………………………………………… 6

本書の構成と使い方 ……………………………………………… 12

▶ Chapter 1　全身状態　General Condition ……………… 16
▶ Chapter 2　外皮　Integument ……………………………… 22
▶ Chapter 3　眼　Eye ……………………………………… 35
▶ Chapter 4　耳　Ear ……………………………………… 44
▶ Chapter 5　鼻　Nose ……………………………………… 47
▶ Chapter 6　呼吸器系　Respiratory System …………… 50
▶ Chapter 7　循環器系　Circulatory System …………… 58
▶ Chapter 8　消化器系　Digestive System ……………… 67
▶ Chapter 9　血液と造血　Blood and Hemopoiesis …… 80
▶ Chapter 10　泌尿器系　Urinary System ………………… 84
▶ Chapter 11　生殖器系　Reproductive System ………… 90
▶ Chapter 12　精神機能　Mental Function ……………… 97
▶ Chapter 13　神経系　Nervous System ………………… 108
▶ Chapter 14　内分泌系と代謝　Endocrine System and Metabolism … 118

英語索引 ……………………………………………………… 122

日本語索引 …………………………………………………… 140

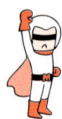

掲載症候（見出し語）一覧

NO.	英語	日本語
Chapter1 全身状態		p.16
001	pyrexia	発熱
002	hypothermia	低体温
003	chill	悪寒
004	short stature	低身長
005	emaciation	やせ
006	obesity	肥満
007	malaise	倦怠感
008	pallor	蒼白
009	convulsion	けいれん
010	vertigo	めまい
011	dehydration	脱水
012	turgor	皮膚緊張度
013	edema	浮腫
014	abscess	膿瘍
015	malformation	奇形
016	shock	ショック
017	sclerosis	硬化
018	atrophy	萎縮
Chapter2 外皮		p.22
019	eruption	発疹
020	macule	斑
021	patch	斑
022	erythema	紅斑
023	purpura	紫斑
024	leukoderma	白斑
025	papule	丘疹
026	nodule	結節
027	tumor	腫瘍
028	vesicle	小水疱
029	bulla	水疱
030	pustule	膿疱
031	cyst	嚢腫
032	wheal	膨疹
033	urticaria	蕁麻疹
034	ulcer	潰瘍
035	erosion	びらん
036	excoriation	表皮剥離
037	fissure	亀裂
038	telangiectasia	毛細血管拡張
039	scale	鱗屑
040	desquamation	落屑
041	acne	痤瘡
042	crust	痂皮
043	keloid	ケロイド
044	gangrene	壊疽
045	enanthema	粘膜疹
046	aphtha	アフタ
047	pruritus	掻痒
048	spoon nail	匙状爪
049	clubbed fingers	ばち指
050	hypertrichosis	多毛症
051	alopecia	脱毛症
052	hyperhidrosis	多汗症
053	night sweat	寝汗
054	seborrhea	脂漏
055	xeroderma	乾皮症
056	jaundice	黄疸
057	vascular spider	くも状血管腫
058	nevus	母斑
059	lymphadenopathy	リンパ節腫脹
060	Virchow's node	ウィルヒョー結節
061	decubitus	褥瘡
062	keratosis	角化症
063	photosensitivity	光線過敏症
Chapter3 眼		p.35
064	refractive error	屈折異常
065	visual field constriction	視野狭窄
066	hemianopia	半盲
067	scotoma	暗点
068	dyschromatopsia	色覚異常

掲載症候（見出し語）一覧

> 本書に収載している症候名の一覧です．
> 語句の発音はダウンロードして聞くことができます（p.14参照）

NO.	英　語	日本語
069	nyctalopia	夜盲症
070	hemeralopia	昼盲症
071	asthenopia	眼精疲労
072	diplopia	複視
073	muscae volitantes	飛蚊症
074	photopsia	光視症
075	metamorphopsia	変視症
076	epiphora	流涙症
077	dry eye	ドライアイ
078	eye mucus	眼脂
079	photophobia	羞明
080	aqueous flare	房水フレア
081	corneal opacity	角膜混濁
082	lens opacity	水晶体混濁
083	leukocoria	白色瞳孔
084	mydriasis	散瞳
085	miosis	縮瞳
086	exophthalmos	眼球突出
087	enophthalmos	眼球陥入
088	blepharoptosis	眼瞼下垂
089	blepharophimosis	瞼裂狭小
090	strabismus	斜視
091	nystagmus	眼振
092	papilledema	乳頭浮腫

Chapter4 耳		p.44
093	conductive hearing loss	伝音難聴
094	sensorineural hearing loss	感音難聴
095	tinnitus	耳鳴り
096	otalgia	耳痛
097	otorrhea	耳漏
098	cerumen	耳垢

Chapter5 鼻		p.47
099	parosmia	嗅覚錯誤
100	saddle nose	鞍鼻

NO.	英　語	日本語
101	nasal obstruction	鼻閉
102	rhinorrhea	鼻漏
103	sneeze	くしゃみ
104	epistaxis	鼻出血
105	nasal polyp	鼻ポリープ

Chapter6 呼吸器系		p.50
106	snore	いびき
107	cough	咳
108	sputum	痰
109	hemoptysis	喀血
110	hoarseness	嗄声
111	pleural effusion	胸水
112	Kussmaul respiration	クスマウル呼吸
113	Cheyne-Stokes respiration	チェーン・ストークス呼吸
114	Biot respiration	ビオー呼吸
115	orthopnea	起坐呼吸
116	prolonged expiration	呼気延長
117	bronchospasm	気管支痙攣
118	coarse crackle	水泡音
119	fine crackle	捻髪音
120	wheeze	喘鳴
121	rhonchus	いびき様音
122	decreased breath sound	呼吸音減弱
123	pleural rub	胸膜摩擦音
124	egophony	山羊声
125	vocal fremitus	声音震盪
126	dyspnea	呼吸困難
127	apnea	無呼吸
128	tachypnea	頻呼吸
129	hyperventilation	過換気

Chapter7 循環器系		p.58
130	third heart sound	Ⅲ音

NO.	英　語	日本語
131	fourth heart sound	Ⅳ音
132	opening snap	開放音
133	midsystolic click	収縮中期クリック
134	gallop rhythm	奔馬調律
135	innocent murmur	無害性雑音
136	systolic ejection murmur	収縮期駆出性雑音
137	pansystolic murmur	汎収縮期雑音
138	diastolic regurgitant murmur	拡張期逆流性雑音
139	middiastolic murmur	拡張中期雑音
140	continuous murmur	連続性雑音
141	pericardial friction rub	心膜摩擦音
142	venous hum	静脈こま音
143	carotid bruit	頸動脈雑音
144	arrhythmia	不整脈
145	tachycardia	頻脈
146	bradycardia	徐脈
147	pulsus celer	速脈
148	pulsus tardus	遅脈
149	alternating pulse	交互脈
150	paradoxical pulse	奇脈
151	palpitation	動悸
152	cardiac arrest	心停止
153	hypertension	高血圧
154	hypotension	低血圧
155	intermittent claudication	間欠性跛行
156	syncope	失神
157	Adams-Stokes syndrome	アダムズ・ストークス症候群
158	cyanosis	チアノーゼ

NO.	英　語	日本語
159	hypoxemia	低酸素血症
160	varicose veins	拡張蛇行静脈
Chapter8 消化器系		**p.67**
161	dysgeusia	味覚異常
162	hyposalivation	唾液分泌不全
163	tongue coating	舌苔
164	strawberry tongue	イチゴ舌
165	macroglossia	巨大舌
166	dental caries	う歯
167	halitosis	口臭
168	fetor hepaticus	肝性口臭
169	trismus	開口障害
170	dysmasesis	咀嚼障害
171	dysphagia	嚥下障害
172	hiccup	しゃっくり
173	pyrosis	胸やけ
174	eructation	おくび
175	flatus	放屁
176	nausea	悪心
177	emesis	嘔吐
178	visceral pain	内臓痛
179	somatic pain	体性痛
180	referred pain	関連痛
181	muscular defense	筋性防御
182	rebound tenderness	反跳圧痛
183	caput medusae	メズサの頭
184	anorexia	食欲不振
185	hyperphagia	過食症
186	dyspepsia	消化不良
187	malabsorption	吸収不良
188	gastric dilatation	胃拡張
189	gastroptosis	胃下垂
190	gastrospasm	胃痙攣
191	hyperchlorhydria	胃酸過多
192	hematemesis	吐血

NO.	英語	日本語
193	hematochezia	鮮血便
194	melena	黒色便
195	acholic stool	無胆汁便
196	diarrhea	下痢
197	constipation	便秘
198	tenesmus	しぶり
199	meteorism	鼓腸
200	borborygmus	腹鳴
201	ascites	腹水
202	hepatomegaly	肝腫大
203	splenomegaly	脾腫
204	abdominal mass	腹部腫瘤

Chapter9 血液と造血　p.80

NO.	英語	日本語
205	anemia	貧血
206	polycythemia	赤血球増加
207	leukocytosis	白血球増加
208	leukemoid reaction	類白血病反応
209	thrombocytopenia	血小板減少
210	hemorrhagic diathesis	出血性素因
211	hypercoagulable state	凝固亢進状態
212	hyperviscosity	過粘稠度

Chapter10 泌尿器系　p.84

NO.	英語	日本語
213	anuria	無尿
214	oliguria	乏尿
215	polyuria	多尿
216	urinary frequency	頻尿
217	nocturia	夜間頻尿
218	dysuria	排尿痛
219	urinary retention	尿閉
220	urinary urgency	尿意切迫
221	urinary incontinence	尿失禁
222	nocturnal enuresis	夜尿症
223	double voiding	二段排尿

NO.	英語	日本語
224	urinary fistula	尿瘻
225	proteinuria	蛋白尿
226	glycosuria	糖尿
227	bilirubinuria	ビリルビン尿
228	hematuria	血尿
229	pyuria	膿尿
230	hemoglobinuria	血色素尿
231	myoglobinuria	ミオグロビン尿
232	chyluria	乳糜尿

Chapter11 生殖器系　p.90

NO.	英語	日本語
233	hematospermia	血精液症
234	uterine prolapse	子宮脱
235	cystocele	膀胱瘤
236	leukorrhea	白帯下
237	dysmenorrhea	月経困難
238	mittelschmerz	中間痛
239	amenorrhea	無月経
240	polymenorrhea	頻発月経
241	oligomenorrhea	希発月経
242	hypermenorrhea	月経過多
243	metrorrhagia	不正子宮出血
244	infertility	不妊
245	hyperemesis gravidarum	妊娠悪阻
246	abortion	流産
247	premature birth	早産
248	precocious puberty	思春期早発症
249	delayed puberty	思春期遅発症
250	premature ejaculation	早漏
251	retrograde ejaculation	逆行性射精
252	erectile dysfunction	勃起不全

NO.	英語	日本語
Chapter12 精神機能		p.97
253	dementia	認知症
254	pseudodementia	仮性認知症
255	amnesia	健忘
256	Korsakoff syndrome	コルサコフ症候群
257	mental retardation	精神遅滞
258	disorientation	見当識障害
259	illusion	錯覚
260	hallucination	幻覚
261	delusion	妄想
262	obsession	強迫
263	anxiety	不安
264	panic attack	パニック発作
265	phobia	恐怖症
266	depressive state	うつ状態
267	manic state	躁状態
268	ambivalence	両価性
269	depersonalization	離人症
270	conversion	転換
271	delusion of control	させられ体験
272	catatonia	緊張病
273	attention deficit hyperactivity disorder (ADHD)	注意欠陥多動性障害
274	distractibility	転導性
275	abulia	無為
276	autism	自閉
277	insomnia	不眠
278	hypersomnia	過眠
279	hypochondriasis	心気症
280	aphasia	失語
281	paraphasia	錯語
282	Broca's aphasia	ブローカ失語
283	Wernicke's aphasia	ウェルニッケ失語
284	apraxia	失行

NO.	英語	日本語
285	agnosia	失認
286	Gerstmann syndrome	ゲルストマン症候群
287	vegetative state	植物状態
288	akinetic mutism	無動無言症
289	locked-in syndrome	閉じ込め症候群
290	somnolence	傾眠
291	stupor	昏迷
292	coma	昏睡
293	delirium	せん妄
294	confusion	錯乱
Chapter13 神経系		p.108
295	Horner syndrome	ホルネル症候群
296	Adie syndrome	アディー症候群
297	Argyll Robertson pupil	アーガイル・ロバートソン瞳孔
298	Bell's palsy	ベル麻痺
299	dysarthria	構音障害
300	Kernig sign	ケルニヒ徴候
301	Brudzinski sign	ブルジンスキー徴候
302	nuchal rigidity	項部硬直
303	megacephaly	大頭症
304	microcephaly	小頭症
305	craniosynostosis	頭蓋縫合早期癒合症
306	spasticity	痙縮
307	Babinski sign	バビンスキー徴候
308	Chaddock reflex	チャドック反射
309	dystonia	ジストニア
310	tremor	振戦
311	chorea	舞踏運動
312	myoclonus	ミオクローヌス
313	ataxia	運動失調
314	Romberg sign	ロンベルク徴候
315	hypesthesia	感覚鈍麻
316	paresthesia	感覚異常

NO.	英語	日本語
317	retropulsion	後方突進
318	orthostatic hypotension	起立性低血圧
319	transverse myelopathy	横断性脊髄症
320	Brown-Sequard syndrome	ブラウン・セカール症候群
321	peripheral neuropathy	末梢神経障害
322	lordosis	前彎
323	kyphosis	後彎
324	scoliosis	側彎
325	ankylosis	関節強直

NO.	英語	日本語
Chapter14　内分泌系と代謝		**p.118**
326	gigantism	巨人症
327	acromegaly	末端肥大症
328	virilism	男性化
329	gynecomastia	女性化乳房
330	goiter	甲状腺腫
331	hyperglycemia	高血糖
332	hyperlipidemia	高脂血症
333	hyperuricemia	高尿酸血症
334	metabolic acidosis	代謝性アシドーシス
335	metabolic alkalosis	代謝性アルカローシス

キャラクター紹介

本書をナビゲートするキャラクター達です

メディカルマン　　　　　ゾーキーズ

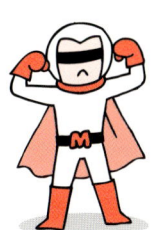

 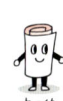 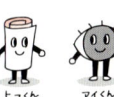

ヒトくん　ヒフくん　アイくん　ミミちゃん　ハナちゃん　ハイくん

 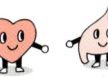 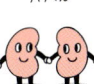

シンちゃん　イーちゃん　チーちゃん　ジンくん　ゾウくん

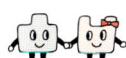 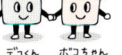

デコくん　ボコちゃん　ノーくん　ロンくん　カンくん

本書の構成と使い方

学習のしかた

1. 本書は14章に分かれていますが、どこから学習を始めても構いません。まず文字で見出し語とその意味、発音記号を確認してから音声を聞き、自分でも発音するようにすると、効果的な学習ができます。

2. 定義を学習する際は、単語1語ずつの意味と文全体の構造が完全に理解できるようになるまで、英文と日本文を何度も見比べてください。

3. 一通り学習したら、見出し語と定義の両方について、英語→日本語、日本語→英語の変換ができるか確認してみてください。定義の日本文全体を英文に変換することが難しい場合は、下線の語だけでも変換できるように頑張ってみてください。

4. 学習を終えたら、チェックボックスにチェックを入れましょう。

❶ 解剖図
Chapterのテーマに関連した解剖図と解剖用語です。

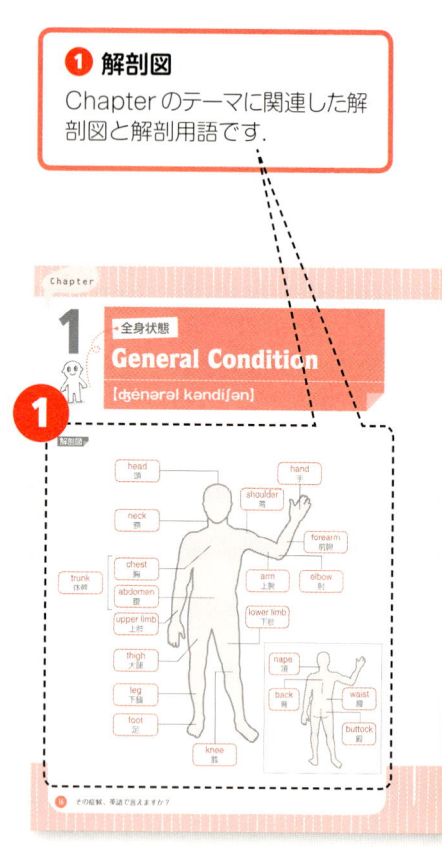

❷ 見出し語

症候名を英語［発音記号］－日本語の順に提示しています．全ての語句についてアメリカ人による発音をダウンロードして聞くことができます．番号は音声のファイル名と対応しています．

（ダウンロードの詳細は「**音声ダウンロードのご案内**」をご覧ください）

❸ 定義

症候の定義を英語と日本語で提示しています．下線の語句は覚えておきたい医学関連用語です．

凡例
- ➡：右の語が左の語の派生語（または関連語）
- ⬅：左の語が右の語の派生語（または関連語）
- ＝：同義語
- ⇔：対義語
- 名：名詞
- 動：動詞
- 形：形容詞

❹ 医学関連用語一覧

Chapterに収載されている医学関連用語を一覧にまとめています．

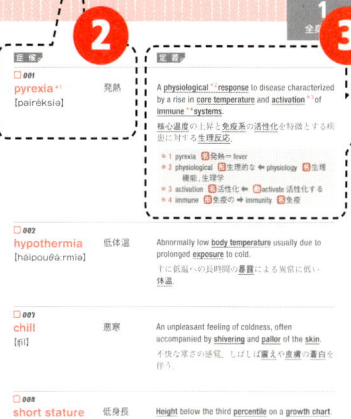

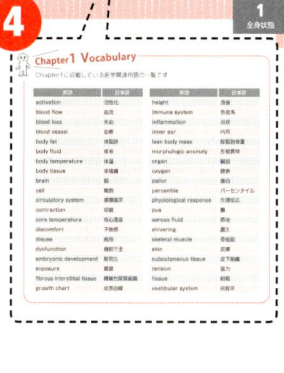

購入者特典

音声ダウンロードのご案内

本書に掲載されている症候の英語名（見出し語）は，羊土社ホームページから音声データをダウンロードして聞くことができます．

ネイティブの発音をくり返し聞いて，耳からの語彙の習得にぜひお役立てください．

・音声データはMP3形式です．MP3形式に対応した標準的なパソコン/オーディオプレーヤーで再生可能です
・ご利用方法など詳細は下記の特典ページをご覧ください

書籍特典利用手順

1 羊土社ホームページにアクセス（下記URL入力または「羊土社」で検索）

http://www.yodosha.co.jp/

2 ［羊土社書籍・雑誌 特典・付録ページ］に移動
羊土社ホームページのトップページに入り口がございます

3 コード入力欄 に下記コードをご入力ください

コード： **ule** - **wslg** - **yxwp** ※すべて半角アルファベット小文字

4 本書特典ページへのリンクが表示されます

※ 羊土社HP会員にご登録いただきますと，2回目以降のご利用の際はコード入力は不要です
※ 羊土社HP会員の詳細につきましては，羊土社HPをご覧ください

その症候、英語で言えますか?

はじめに覚える335症候と
ついでに覚える1000の関連語

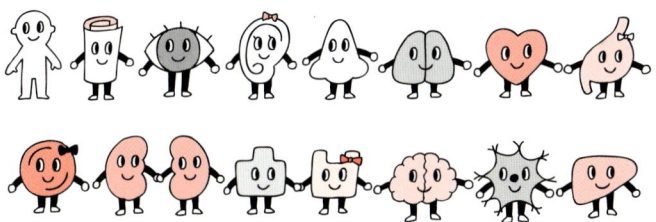

Chapter

1

全身状態
General Condition
【ʤénərəl kəndíʃən】

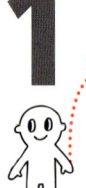

解剖図

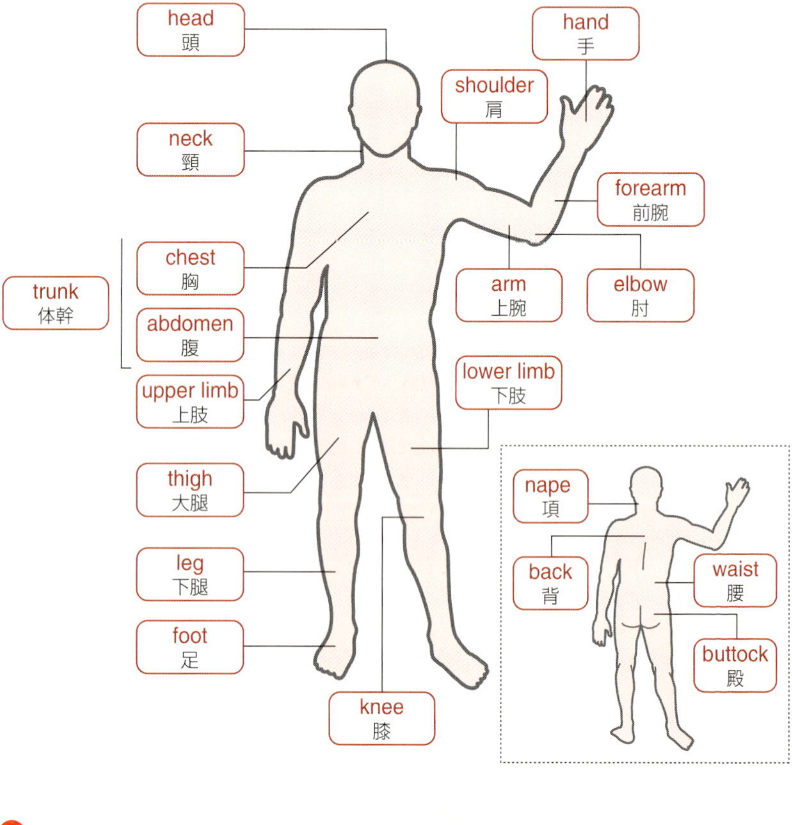

- head 頭
- hand 手
- shoulder 肩
- neck 頸
- forearm 前腕
- trunk 体幹
  - chest 胸
  - abdomen 腹
- arm 上腕
- elbow 肘
- upper limb 上肢
- lower limb 下肢
- thigh 大腿
- nape 項
- leg 下腿
- back 背
- waist 腰
- foot 足
- buttock 殿
- knee 膝

その症候、英語で言えますか？

1 全身状態

症候		定義

001
pyrexia[*1] 発熱
【pairéksiə】

A **physiological**[*2] **response** to disease characterized by a rise in **core temperature** and **activation**[*3] of **immune**[*4] **systems**.

核心温度の上昇と免疫系の活性化を特徴とする疾患に対する生理反応.

- *1 pyrexia 名発熱= fever
- *2 physiological 形生理的な ← physiology 名生理機能,生理学
- *3 activation 名活性化 ← 動activate 活性化する
- *4 immune 形免疫の → immunity 名免疫

002
hypothermia 低体温
【hàipouθə́:rmiə】

Abnormally low **body temperature** usually due to prolonged **exposure** to cold.

主に低温への長時間の暴露による異常に低い体温.

003
chill 悪寒
【tʃíl】

An unpleasant feeling of coldness, often accompanied by **shivering** and **pallor** of the **skin**.

不快な寒さの感覚.しばしば震えや皮膚の蒼白を伴う.

004
short stature 低身長
【ʃɔ́:rt stǽtʃər】

Height below the third **percentile** on a **growth chart**.

成長曲線上で3パーセンタイル未満の身長.

症候		定義

005
emaciation やせ
[iméiʃiéiʃən]

Extreme loss of <u>body fat</u> and <u>lean body mass</u>, usually applied to a BMI under 18.5.

<u>体脂肪</u>と<u>除脂肪体重</u>の極端な減少．通常はBMIが18.5未満をいう．

006
obesity 肥満
[oubí:səti]

An excess of <u>body fat</u> in comparison to <u>lean body mass</u>, usually applied to a BMI over 25.

<u>除脂肪体重</u>に比較して<u>体脂肪</u>が過剰な状態．通常はBMIが25以上をいう．

007
malaise 倦怠感
[mæléiz]

A vague bodily <u>discomfort</u> due to the metabolic[*1] alterations caused by illness.

疾患による代謝の変化に起因する漠然とした全身の<u>不快感</u>．

[*1] metabolic 形代謝の ← metabolism 名代謝

008
pallor 蒼白
[pǽlər]

Abnormal paleness of the <u>skin</u> due to decreased <u>blood flow</u>.

<u>血流</u>の減少による<u>皮膚</u>の異常な青白さ．

009
convulsion けいれん
[kənvʌ́lʃən]

Involuntary[*1] <u>contractions</u>[*2] of <u>skeletal muscles</u> due to abnormal electrical activity in the <u>brain</u>.

脳の異常な電気活動による<u>骨格筋</u>の不随意な<u>収縮</u>．

[*1] involuntary 形不随意の ⟷ voluntary 形随意の
[*2] contraction 名収縮 ← contract 動収縮する

1 全身状態

症候 / 定義

010
vertigo
【və́:rtigòu】
めまい
A sensation of spinning due to **dysfunction** of the **vestibular**[*1] **system** in the **inner ear**.
内耳の前庭系の機能不全による目がまわる感覚.

* 1 vestibular 形 前庭の ← vestibule 名 前庭

011
dehydration
【dì:haidréiʃən】
脱水
Excessive loss of water or **body fluids**.
水分または体液の過度の減少.

012
turgor
【tə́:rgər】
皮膚緊張度
The normal **tension** of the **skin** maintained by the fluid content of **blood vessels** and **cells**.
血管や細胞の水分量により保たれる正常な皮膚の張力.

013
edema
【idí:mə】
浮腫
An excessive accumulation of **serous**[*1] **fluid** in the **subcutaneous**[*2] **tissues**.
皮下組織における漿液の過剰な貯留.

* 1 serous 形 漿液(性)の ← serum 名 漿液
* 2 subcutaneous 形 皮下の ← cutaneous 形 皮膚の ← cutis 名 皮膚

014
abscess
【ǽbses】
膿瘍
A localized[*1] collection of **pus** frequently associated with **inflammation**.
しばしば炎症に関連する膿の局在性集積.

* 1 localized 形 局在性の

症候		定義

015
malformation 奇形
【mælfɔ:rméiʃən】

A congenital[*1] morphologic[*2] anomaly[*3] resulting from errors in embryonic[*4] development.

胚発生中の欠陥に起因する先天性形態異常.

- *1 congenital 形 先天性の
- *2 morphologic 形 形態の，形態学的な
  ← morphology 名 形態学
- *3 anomaly 名 異常, 奇形
- *4 embryonic 形 胚の ← embryo 名 胚

016
shock ショック
【ʃák】

Inadequate supply of oxygen to body tissues due to failure of the circulatory system or blood loss.

循環器系の障害または失血による体組織への不十分な酸素の供給.

017
sclerosis 硬化
【skliróusis】

Hardening or thickening of body tissues, as by excessive formation of fibrous interstitial[*1] tissue.

線維性間質組織の過剰形成などにより体組織が硬くなる，もしくは肥厚すること.

- *1 interstitial 形 間質の ← interstitium 名 間質

018
atrophy 萎縮
【ǽtrəfi】

A decrease in size of an organ or tissue caused by disease or disuse.

疾患または廃用に起因する臓器または組織の縮小.

1 全身状態

Chapter 1 Vocabulary

Chapter1に収載している医学関連用語の一覧です

英語	日本語	英語	日本語
activation	活性化	height	身長
blood flow	血流	immune system	免疫系
blood loss	失血	inflammation	炎症
blood vessel	血管	inner ear	内耳
body fat	体脂肪	lean body mass	除脂肪体重
body fluid	体液	morphologic anomaly	形態異常
body temperature	体温	organ	臓器
body tissue	体組織	oxygen	酸素
brain	脳	pallor	蒼白
cell	細胞	percentile	パーセンタイル
circulatory system	循環器系	physiological response	生理反応
contraction	収縮	pus	膿
core temperature	核心温度	serous fluid	漿液
discomfort	不快感	shivering	震え
disuse	廃用	skeletal muscle	骨格筋
dysfunction	機能不全	skin	皮膚
embryonic development	胚発生	subcutaneous tissue	皮下組織
exposure	暴露	tension	張力
fibrous interstitial tissue	線維性間質組織	tissue	組織
growth chart	成長曲線	vestibular system	前庭系

Chapter 2

外皮
Integument
【intégjumənt】

解剖図

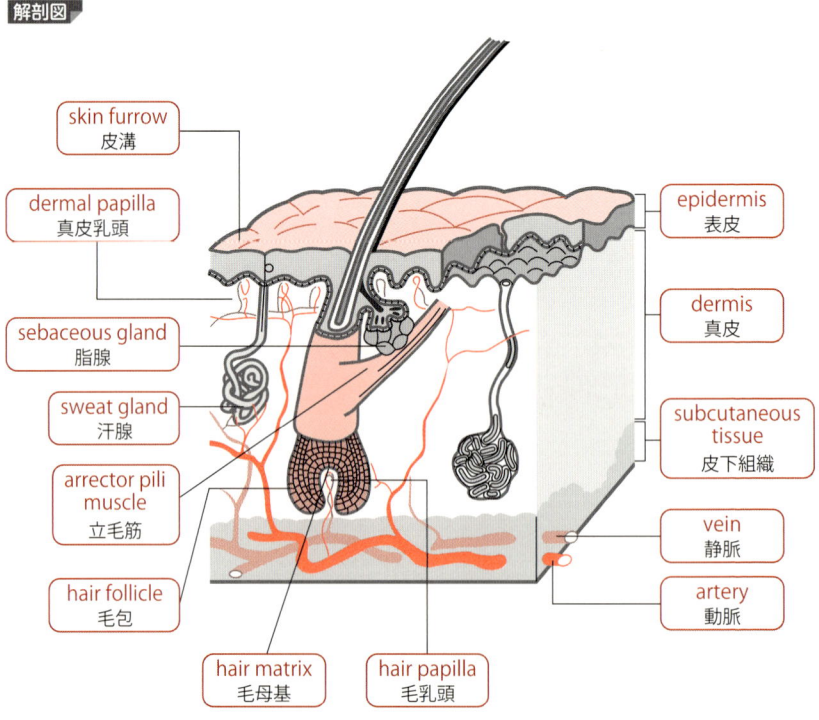

2 外皮

症候 | **定義**

019
eruption*¹
【irʌ́pʃən】
発疹

A rapidly developing **lesion** of the **skin** with altered color or texture.

急速に形成される<u>皮膚</u>の<u>病変</u>で，色や手ざわりの変化を伴う．

*1 eruption 名 発疹＝rash

020
macule
【mǽkjuːl】
斑

A flat, discolored*¹ area on the skin up to 1 cm in diameter.

皮膚上の扁平な変色部分で直径1cmまでのもの．

*1 discolored 形 変色した

021
patch
【pǽtʃ】
斑

A flat, discolored area on the skin more than 1 cm in diameter.

皮膚上の扁平な変色部分で直径1cmを超えるもの．

022
erythema
【èrəθíːmə】
紅斑

Redness of the skin due to **dilation***¹ or **congestion** of the **capillaries**.

<u>毛細血管</u>の<u>拡張</u>や<u>うっ血</u>による皮膚の赤み．

*1 dilation 名 拡張 ← dilate 動 拡張する

023
purpura
【pə́ːrpjurə】
紫斑

Purplish spots on the skin caused by **subcutaneous hemorrhage**.

<u>皮下出血</u>に起因する皮膚上の紫色の斑点．

症候		定義

☐ 024
leukoderma 白斑
【lùːkədə́ːrmə】

Partial or total loss of skin **pigmentation**.
皮膚の**色素沈着**の部分的または完全な欠如.

☐ 025
papule 丘疹
【pǽpjuːl】

A circumscribed*¹, solid*² **elevation** of the skin up to 1 cm in diameter.
皮膚の限局性，充実性**隆起**で直径1cmまでのもの.

* 1 circumscribed 形 限局性の
* 2 solid 形 充実性の

☐ 026
nodule 結節
【nɑ́dʒuːl】

A circumscribed, solid **elevation** of the skin more than 1 cm in diameter.
皮膚の限局性，充実性**隆起**で直径1cmを超えるもの.

☐ 027
tumor 腫瘍
【t(j)úːmər】

Abnormal mass of rapidly proliferating*¹ cells that may be benign*² or malignant*³.
急速に増殖する細胞の異常な塊で，良性または悪性に分けられる.

* 1 proliferate 動 増殖する ➡ proliferation 名 増殖
* 2 benign 形 良性の
* 3 malignant 形 悪性の

2 外皮

症候 | **定義**

□ 028
vesicle
【vésikl】
小水疱

A circumscribed **elevation** of the skin up to 1 cm in diameter containing watery fluid.

水様の液体を含む皮膚の限局性**隆起**で直径1cmまでのもの.

□ 029
bulla
【búlə】
水疱

A circumscribed **elevation** of the skin more than 1 cm in diameter containing watery fluid.

水様の液体を含む皮膚の限局性**隆起**で直径1cmを超えるもの.

□ 030
pustule
【pʌ́stʃuːl】
膿疱

A circumscribed **elevation** of the skin containing purulent[*1] **exudates**.

膿性**滲出物**を含む皮膚の限局性**隆起**.

* 1 purulent 形 膿性の, 化膿性の ← purulence 名 膿, 化膿

□ 031
cyst
【síst】
嚢腫

An abnormal membranous[*1] **sac** containing gas, fluid, or cellular[*2] substance.

気体, 液体, または細胞性物質を含む異常な膜性の**嚢**.

* 1 membranous 形 膜性の ← membrane 名 膜
* 2 cellular 形 細胞の ← cell 名 細胞

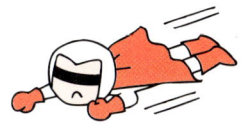

症候		定義

032
wheal 膨疹
【wiːl】

A circumscribed, transient <u>elevation</u> of the skin caused by <u>edema</u> of the <u>dermis</u>.

<u>真皮</u>の<u>浮腫</u>に起因する皮膚の限局性，一過性<u>隆起</u>．

033
urticaria[*1] 蕁麻疹
【əːrtəkæriə】

An <u>allergic</u>[*2] <u>reaction</u> characterized by the development of <u>wheals</u> and intense <u>itching</u>.

膨疹の発生と強いかゆみを特徴とする<u>アレルギー反応</u>．

* 1 urticaria 名 蕁麻疹 = hives
* 2 allergic 形 アレルギーの ← allergy 名 アレルギー

034
ulcer 潰瘍
【ʌ́lsər】

A <u>lesion</u> of the skin or a <u>mucous membrane</u> accompanied by formation of <u>pus</u> and loss of surrounding <u>tissue</u>.

膿の形成と周辺<u>組織</u>の欠損を伴う皮膚または<u>粘膜</u>の<u>病変</u>．

035
erosion びらん
【iróuʒən】

A superficial <u>ulcer</u> with <u>tissue loss</u> in the <u>epidermis</u> or <u>mucosa</u>.

<u>表皮</u>または粘膜の<u>組織欠損</u>を伴う表層の<u>潰瘍</u>．

2 外皮

症候		定義

036
excoriation *1
【ikskɔ̀:riéiʃən】

表皮剥離

Circumscribed removal of the superficial layers of skin or **mucous membrane**.

皮膚や**粘膜**の表層の限局性欠損.

* 1 excoriation 名 表皮剥離＝ abrasion 名 擦過傷

037
fissure
【fíʃər】

亀裂

A deep linear split in the skin reaching into the **dermis**.

真皮にまで達する皮膚の深い線状の切れ目.

038
telangiectasia
【tilændʒiektéiʒə】

毛細血管拡張

Chronic *1 **dilation** of **capillaries** causing red spots or branching lines on the skin.

皮膚上に赤い斑点や分枝した線を形成する**毛細血管**の慢性の**拡張**.

* 1 chronic 形 慢性の ⇔ acute 形 急性の

039
scale *1
【skéil】

鱗屑

Cornified *2 **epidermal** *3 **cells** forming flakes on the skin surface.

皮膚表面で薄片を形成する角化した**表皮細胞**.

* 1 scale 名 鱗屑＝ squama
* 2 cornified 形 角化した ➡ cornification 名 角化
* 3 epidermal 形 表皮の ⬅ epidermis 名 表皮

040
desquamation
【dìskwəméiʃən】

落屑

The shedding of the superficial **epithelium** of the skin as **scales**.

皮膚の表層**上皮**が**鱗屑**となって脱落すること.

症候		定義

041
acne　痤瘡
【ǽkni】

An inflammatory*¹ disease of <u>sebaceous glands</u> and <u>hair follicles</u> that is marked by <u>papules</u> or <u>pustules</u>.

<u>脂腺</u>および<u>毛包</u>の炎症性疾患で，<u>丘疹</u>または<u>膿疱</u>を伴う．

＊1 inflammatory 形 炎症性の ← inflammation 名 炎症

042
crust　痂皮
【krʌ́st】

Dried <u>deposit</u> of blood or <u>pus</u> covering the surface of an <u>abrasion</u> or a ruptured <u>vesicle</u>, <u>bulla</u>, or <u>pustule</u>.

<u>擦過傷</u>または破れた<u>小水疱</u>，<u>水疱</u>，膿疱の表面を覆う乾燥した血液や膿の<u>沈着物</u>．

043
keloid　ケロイド
【kíːlɔid】

An elevated, enlarging, firm <u>scar tissue</u> consisting of irregularly distributed bands of <u>collagen</u>.

隆起し拡大する硬い<u>瘢痕組織</u>で，不規則に分布する<u>コラーゲン</u>の束から形成される．

044
gangrene　壊疽
【gǽŋgriːn】

Death of <u>tissue</u> associated with lack of <u>blood supply</u> and bacterial <u>infection</u>.

<u>血液供給</u>の欠如および細菌<u>感染</u>に関連する<u>組織</u>の死．

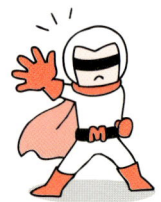

その症候、英語で言えますか？

2 外皮

症候		定義

□ *045*

enanthema
【ènænθíːma】

粘膜疹

An **eruption** on a **mucous membrane** such as the **oral mucosa** and **external genitalia**[*1].
口腔粘膜や外陰部などの粘膜に生じる発疹.

* 1 genitalia 名 生殖器（複数形；通常は複数形を使用する）

□ *046*

aphtha
【ǽfθə】

アフタ

A small, round **ulcer** on the **oral mucosa** terminating in a white **slough**.
口腔粘膜に生じる小さい円形の潰瘍で，最終的に白い脱落組織となる.

□ *047*

pruritus
【pruráitəs】

掻痒

Localized or generalized[*1] **itching** due to **irritation** of **sensory nerve**[*2] **endings**[*3].
感覚神経終末の刺激による局在性または全身性のかゆみ.

* 1 generalized 形 全身性の
* 2 sensory nerve 名 感覚神経
* 3 nerve ending 名 神経終末

□ *048*

spoon nail
【spúːn néil】

匙状爪

Abnormal **concavity** of **nails** associated with **iron deficiency**[*1] or occupational contact with **chemicals**.
鉄欠乏または職業上の化学物質との接触と関連する爪の異常な陥凹.

* 1 deficiency 名 欠乏

症候	定義

☐ 049
clubbed fingers ばち指
【klʌ́bd fíŋgərz】

Thickening and widening of the <u>extremities</u> of the fingers due to <u>proliferation</u> of <u>nail bed</u> tissues.
<u>爪床</u>組織の<u>増殖</u>により指の<u>末端</u>が厚く幅広くなること．

☐ 050
hypertrichosis 多毛症
【háipərtrikóusis】

Abnormal increase in hair growth caused by increased <u>androgen</u> secretion, <u>drugs</u>, or <u>starvation</u>.
アンドロゲン分泌の亢進，<u>薬物</u>，または<u>飢餓</u>に起因する毛の成長の異常な亢進．

☐ 051
alopecia 脱毛症
【æ̀ləpíːsiə】

Abnormal <u>hair loss</u> caused by primary [*1] <u>cutaneous disorders</u>, <u>drugs</u>, or <u>systemic</u> [*2] <u>diseases</u>.
<u>原発性</u><u>皮膚疾患</u>，<u>薬物</u>，または<u>全身性疾患</u>に起因する異常な<u>脱毛</u>．

*1 primary 形 原発性の
*2 systemic 形 全身性の

☐ 052
hyperhidrosis 多汗症
【háipərhidróusis】

Localized or generalized excessive <u>perspiration</u>. [*1]
局在性または全身性の過剰な<u>発汗</u>．

*1 perspiration 名 発汗 = sweating

☐ 053
night sweat 寝汗
【náit swét】

Profuse <u>perspiration</u> during sleep, often associated with <u>tuberculosis</u> or <u>menopause</u>.
睡眠中の多量の<u>発汗</u>．しばしば<u>結核</u>や<u>閉経</u>と関連する．

症候		定義

☐ 054
seborrhea 脂漏
【sèbərí:ə】

Overactivity of the <u>sebaceous glands</u>, resulting in an excessive amount of <u>sebum</u>.

<u>脂腺</u>の過活動による<u>皮脂</u>の過剰.

☐ 055
xeroderma 乾皮症
【zìrədé:rmə】

Excessive dryness of the skin due to diminished <u>secretion</u> of <u>sebum</u> and <u>sweat</u>.

<u>皮脂</u>および<u>汗</u>の<u>分泌</u>の減少による皮膚の過剰な乾燥.

☐ 056
jaundice 黄疸
【dʒɔ́:ndis】

Yellow <u>discoloration</u> of the skin and eyes due to elevated <u>blood levels</u> of bilirubin.

ビリルビンの<u>血中濃度</u>の上昇による皮膚および眼の黄色い<u>変色</u>.

☐ 057
vascular spider＊¹ くも状血管腫
【væskjulər spáidər】

An <u>angioma</u> with radiating <u>capillary</u> branches found slightly below the skin surface.

放射状の<u>毛細血管</u>の枝をもつ<u>血管腫</u>で，皮下浅層にみられる.

＊1 vascular spider 名 くも状血管腫＝ spider angioma

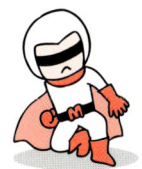

症候		定義

☐ 058

nevus
【níːvəs】

母斑

A circumscribed **malformation** of the skin colored by **hyperpigmentation**[*1] or increased **vascularity**.

色素沈着過剰や血管分布の増加により色を呈する皮膚の限局性奇形.

- [*1] hyperpigmentation 名 色素沈着過剰
  ← pigmentation 名 色素沈着

☐ 059

lymphadenopathy
【limfædənápəθi】

リンパ節
腫脹

An abnormal **swelling** of **lymph nodes** usually associated with **infection** or **tumor**.

リンパ節の異常な腫れで,通常は感染または腫瘍と関連する.

☐ 060

Virchow's node[*1]
【fíərkouz nóud】

ウィルヒョー結節

A swollen **lymph node** in the left **supraclavicular fossa** that indicates the presence of **cancer** in the **abdominal cavity**.

左鎖骨上窩の腫脹したリンパ節で,腹腔内の癌の存在を示唆する.

- [*1] Virchow's node 名 ウィルヒョー結節
  ＝ signal node 名 警報リンパ節

☐ 061

decubitus[*1]
【dikjúːbitəs】

褥瘡

An **ulceration** of **tissue** caused by lack of **blood supply** due to prolonged pressure.

長時間の圧迫による血液供給の欠如に起因する組織の潰瘍化.

- [*1] decubitus 名 褥瘡 ＝ bedsore 名 床ずれ

2 外皮

症候 / 定義

☐ **062**

keratosis 角化症
【kèrətóusis】

A skin <u>lesion</u> characterized by <u>overgrowth</u> and thickening of the <u>cornified epithelium</u>.
<u>角化上皮</u>の<u>過形成</u>および肥厚を特徴とする皮膚<u>病変</u>.

☐ **063**

photosensitivity 光線過敏症
【fòutousènsətívəti】

An abnormal cutaneous response to <u>sunlight</u> or <u>ultraviolet radiation</u> caused by certain disorders or <u>drugs</u>.
特定の疾患や<u>薬物</u>に起因する<u>日光</u>や<u>紫外線</u>に対する異常な皮膚の反応.

Chapter 2 Vocabulary

Chapter2に収載している医学関連用語の一覧です

英語	日本語	英語	日本語
abdominal cavity	腹腔	collagen	コラーゲン
abrasion	擦過傷	concavity	陥凹
allergic reaction	アレルギー反応	congestion	うっ血
androgen	アンドロゲン	cornified epithelium	角化上皮
angioma	血管腫	cutaneous disorder	皮膚疾患
bilirubin	ビリルビン	deposit	沈着物
blood level	血中濃度	dermis	真皮
blood supply	血液供給	dilation	拡張
bulla	水疱	discoloration	変色
cancer	癌	drug	薬物
capillary	毛細血管	edema	浮腫
chemical	化学物質	elevation	隆起

33

英語	日本語	英語	日本語
epidermal cell	表皮細胞	pus	膿
epidermis	表皮	pustule	膿疱
epithelium	上皮	sac	嚢
eruption	発疹	scale	鱗屑
external genitalia	外陰部	scar tissue	瘢痕組織
extremity	末端	sebaceous gland	脂腺
exudate	滲出物	sebum	皮脂
hair follicle	毛包	secretion	分泌
hair loss	脱毛	sensory nerve ending	感覚神経終末
hyperpigmentation	色素沈着過剰	skin	皮膚
infection	感染	slough	脱落組織
iron deficiency	鉄欠乏	starvation	飢餓
irritation	刺激	subcutaneous hemorrhage	皮下出血
itching	かゆみ	sunlight	日光
lesion	病変	supraclavicular fossa	鎖骨上窩
lymph node	リンパ節	sweat	汗
malformation	奇形	swelling	腫れ
menopause	閉経	systemic disease	全身性疾患
mucosa	粘膜	tissue	組織
mucous membrane	粘膜	tissue loss	組織欠損
nail	爪	tuberculosis	結核
nail bed	爪床	tumor	腫瘍
oral mucosa	口腔粘膜	ulcer	潰瘍
overgrowth	過形成	ulceration	潰瘍化
papule	丘疹	ultraviolet radiation	紫外線
perspiration	発汗	vascularity	血管分布
pigmentation	色素沈着	vesicle	小水疱
proliferation	増殖	wheal	膨疹

Chapter 3

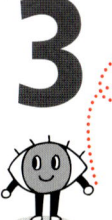

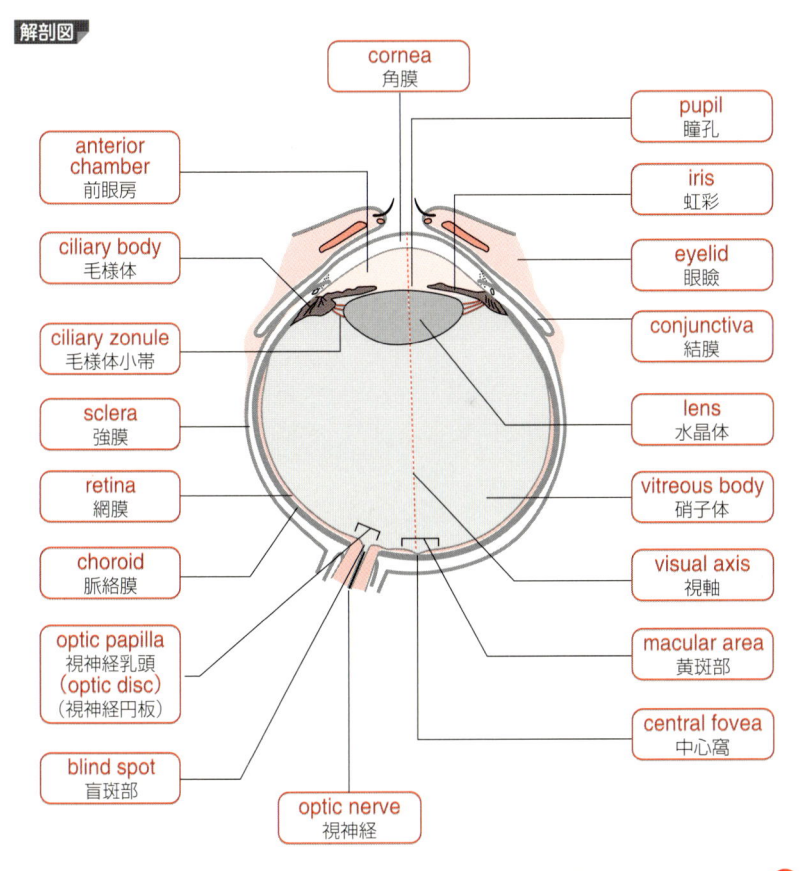

眼
Eye
【ái】

解剖図

- cornea 角膜
- pupil 瞳孔
- anterior chamber 前眼房
- iris 虹彩
- ciliary body 毛様体
- eyelid 眼瞼
- ciliary zonule 毛様体小帯
- conjunctiva 結膜
- sclera 強膜
- lens 水晶体
- retina 網膜
- vitreous body 硝子体
- choroid 脈絡膜
- visual axis 視軸
- optic papilla 視神経乳頭 (optic disc)（視神経円板）
- macular area 黄斑部
- central fovea 中心窩
- blind spot 盲斑部
- optic nerve 視神経

症候		定義

☐ 064
refractive error[*1]
【rifræktiv érər】

屈折異常

The inability of the lens of the eye to focus light rays correctly on the retina.

眼の水晶体が網膜に光線の焦点を正確に合わせられない状態.

*1 refractive 形 屈折の ← refraction 名 屈折

☐ 065
visual field constriction
【víʒuəl fíːld kənstríkʃən】

視野狭窄

Loss of vision in the peripheral[*1] visual field.

周辺視野における視力の喪失.

*1 peripheral 形 周辺の, 末梢の ← periphery 名 周辺, 末梢

☐ 066
hemianopia
【hemiənóupiə】

半盲

Loss of vision in one half of the visual field of one or both eyes.

片目または両目の視野の半分における視力の喪失.

☐ 067
scotoma
【skoutóumə】

暗点

An area of decreased or lost vision within the visual field.

視野の内部で視力が低下または失われた部分.

☐ 068
dyschromatopsia
【diskroumətápsiə】

色覚異常

Abnormal color perception due to absence or deficiency of cone pigments in the retina.

網膜の錐体色素の欠損または障害による異常な色覚.

3 眼

| 症 候 | | 定 義 |

□ *069*

nyctalopia **1*　　夜盲症
[nìktəlóupiə]

Reduced **visual acuity** in faint light due to impaired **rod** function.
<u>杆体</u>機能の障害による薄明りでの<u>視力</u>の低下．

＊1　nyctalopia 名 夜盲症＝night blindness

□ *070*

hemeralopia **1*　　昼盲症
[hèmərəlóupiə]

Reduced **visual acuity** in bright light due to impaired **cone** function.
<u>錐体</u>機能の障害による明るい光の中での<u>視力</u>の低下．

＊1　hemeralopia 名 昼盲症＝day blindness

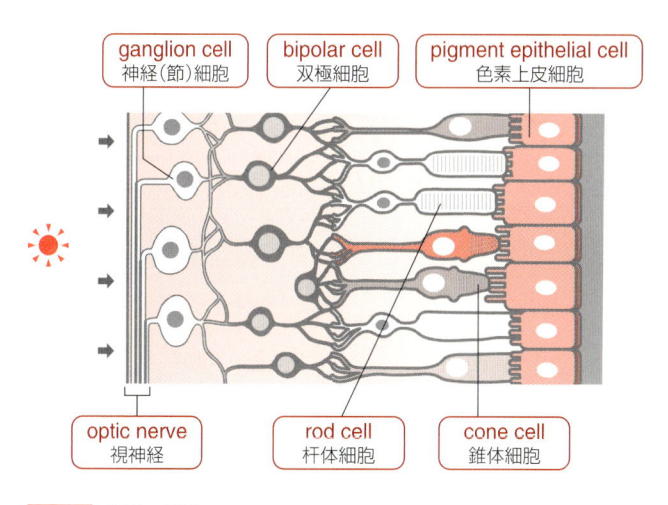

ganglion cell
神経(節)細胞

bipolar cell
双極細胞

pigment epithelial cell
色素上皮細胞

optic nerve
視神経

rod cell
杆体細胞

cone cell
錐体細胞

解剖図　網膜の構造

| 症　候 | | 定　義 |

071
asthenopia　眼精疲労
【æsθənóupiə】

Fatigue of the eyes often accompanied by **eye pain**, **headache**, and **blurred vision**.
眼痛，頭痛，かすみ目をしばしば伴う眼の疲労．

072
diplopia[*1]　複視
【diplóupiə】

The simultaneous perception of two images of a single object.
単一の物体に対して2つの像を同時に知覚すること．

*1 diplopia 名 複視＝double vision

073
muscae volitantes　飛蚊症
【mʌ́ski: valitǽntiz】

Appearance of moving spots before the eyes due to **cell fragments** in the **vitreous humor**.
硝子体液中の細胞断片により眼前に動く点が現れること．

074
photopsia　光視症
【foutápsiə】

A subjective sensation of lights, sparks, or colors due to electrical or mechanical **stimulation** of the **ocular**[*1] **system**.
視覚系の電気的または機械的刺激により光，閃光，色を主観的に知覚すること．

*1 ocular 形 視覚の，眼の ← oculus 名 眼

075
metamorphopsia　変視症
【metəmɔ:fápsiə】

A **visual disturbance** in which objects appear to be distorted.
物体が歪んで見える視覚障害．

症候		定義

076
epiphora 流涙症
【ipífərə】

An overflow of tears due to excessive tear <u>secretion</u> or <u>obstruction</u> of the <u>lacrimal</u>*¹ <u>passages</u>.
過剰な涙の<u>分泌</u>または<u>涙道</u>の<u>閉塞</u>による涙の流漏.

*1 lacrimal 形 涙の

077
dry eye ドライアイ
【drái ái】

<u>Corneal</u>*¹ dryness due to deficient tear production.
涙の産出不足による角膜の乾燥.

*1 corneal 形 角膜の ← cornea 名 角膜

078
eye mucus 眼脂
【ái mjúːkəs】

A <u>mucous</u>*¹ substance discharged from the ocular surface.
眼表面から排出される粘液性の物質.

*1 mucous 形 粘液性の ← mucus 名 粘液

079
photophobia 羞明
【fòutəfóubiə】

Experience of <u>discomfort</u> or pain to the eyes due to light <u>exposure</u>.
光への<u>暴露</u>により眼に<u>不快感</u>や痛みを経験すること.

080
aqueous flare 房水フレア
【éikwiəs fléər】

<u>Turbidity</u>*¹ of <u>aqueous humor</u> due to leakage of <u>protein</u> into the <u>anterior chamber</u>.
<u>前眼房</u>への<u>蛋白</u>の漏入による<u>眼房水</u>の<u>混濁</u>.

*1 turbidity 名 混濁 ← turbid 形 混濁した

症候		定義

☐ *081*
corneal opacity 角膜混濁
【kó:niəl oupǽsəti】

Clouding in the central or peripheral area of the <u>cornea</u> caused by <u>infection</u> or injury.

<u>感染</u>または外傷に起因する<u>角膜</u>中心部または周辺部の濁り．

☐ *082*
lens opacity 水晶体混濁
【lénz oupǽsəti】

Clouding of the <u>lens</u> that obstructs the passage of light and causes partial or total <u>blindness</u>.

光の通過を妨げ，部分的または完全な<u>失明</u>を引き起こす<u>水晶体</u>の濁り．

☐ *083*
leukocoria 白色瞳孔
【lu:koukó:riə】

Abnormal reflection from the <u>retina</u> giving the appearance of a white <u>pupil</u>.

<u>瞳孔</u>を白く見せる<u>網膜</u>からの異常な反射．

☐ *084*
mydriasis 散瞳
【midráiəsis】

Pupillary *¹ <u>dilation</u> caused by <u>contraction</u> of the <u>dilator muscle</u> of the <u>iris</u>.

<u>虹彩</u>の<u>散大筋</u>の<u>収縮</u>による瞳孔の<u>拡張</u>．

＊1 pupillary 形 瞳孔の ← pupil 名 瞳孔

☐ *085*
miosis 縮瞳
【maióusis】

Pupillary <u>constriction</u> caused by <u>contraction</u> of the <u>sphincter muscle</u> of the <u>iris</u>.

<u>虹彩</u>の<u>括約筋</u>の<u>収縮</u>による瞳孔の<u>縮小</u>．

3 眼

症候 / 定義

☐ *086*
exophthalmos 眼球突出
【eksɑfθǽləməs】

Abnormal **protrusion**[*1] of the **eyeball** from the **orbit**.
眼窩からの眼球の異常な突出.

* 1 protrusion 名 突出 ⬅ protrude 動 突出する

☐ *087*
enophthalmos 眼球陥入
【inɑfθǽləməs】

Abnormal **recession** of the **eyeball** within the **orbit**.
眼窩内への眼球の異常な陥入.

☐ *088*
blepharoptosis 眼瞼下垂
【blefəroutóusis】

Drooping or abnormal **relaxation** of the **upper eyelid**[*1].
上眼瞼の垂れ下がりまたは異常な弛緩.

* 1 upper eyelid 名 上眼瞼 ⬌ lower eyelid 名 下眼瞼

☐ *089*
blepharophimosis 瞼裂狭小
【blefəroufaimóusis】

Horizontal and vertical narrowing of the **palpebral**[*1] **fissure**.
眼瞼裂の水平方向および垂直方向の狭小.

* 1 palpebral 形 眼瞼の ⬅ palpebra 名 眼瞼

☐ *090*
strabismus 斜視
【strəbízməs】

A constant lack of parallelism of the **visual axes**[*1] of the eyes.
両目の視軸の平行を常に欠いている状態.

* 1 visual axes 名 視軸（複数形；単数形は visual axis）

症候		定義

☐ 091

nystagmus 眼振 Involuntary rhythmic <u>oscillation</u> of the <u>eyeballs</u>.
【nistǽgməs】 <u>眼球</u>の不随意性で律動性の<u>振動</u>.

☐ 092

papilledema 乳頭浮腫 <u>Edema</u> of the <u>optic disc</u>, often due to increased
【pəpilidí:mə】 <u>intracranial</u>*¹ <u>pressure</u>.
<u>視神経円板</u>の<u>浮腫</u>. しばしば<u>頭蓋内圧</u>の上昇による.

> *1 intracranial 形 頭蓋内の ← cranial 形 頭蓋の ← cranium 名 頭蓋

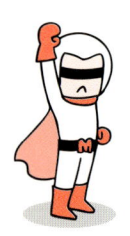

Chapter 3 Vocabulary

Chapter3に収載している医学関連用語の一覧です

英語	日本語	英語	日本語
anterior chamber	前眼房	obstruction	閉塞
aqueous humor	眼房水	ocular system	視覚系
blindness	失明	optic disc	視神経円板
blurred vision	かすみ目	orbit	眼窩
cell fragment	細胞断片	oscillation	振動
color perception	色覚	palpebral fissure	眼瞼裂
cone	錐体	peripheral visual field	周辺視野
cone pigment	錐体色素	protein	蛋白
constriction	縮小	protrusion	突出
contraction	収縮	pupil	瞳孔
cornea	角膜	recession	陥入
dilation	拡張	relaxation	弛緩
dilator muscle	散大筋	retina	網膜
discomfort	不快感	rod	杆体
edema	浮腫	secretion	分泌
exposure	暴露	sphincter muscle	括約筋
eye pain	眼痛	stimulation	刺激
eyeball	眼球	turbidity	混濁
fatigue	疲労	upper eyelid	上眼瞼
headache	頭痛	vision	視力
infection	感染	visual acuity	視力
intracranial pressure	頭蓋内圧	visual axes (visual axis)	視軸
iris	虹彩	visual disturbance	視覚障害
lacrimal passage	涙道	visual field	視野
lens	水晶体	vitreous humor	硝子体液

Chapter

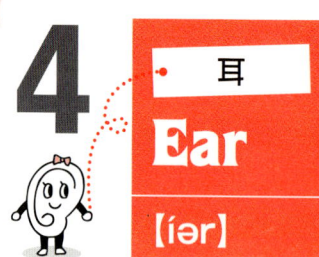

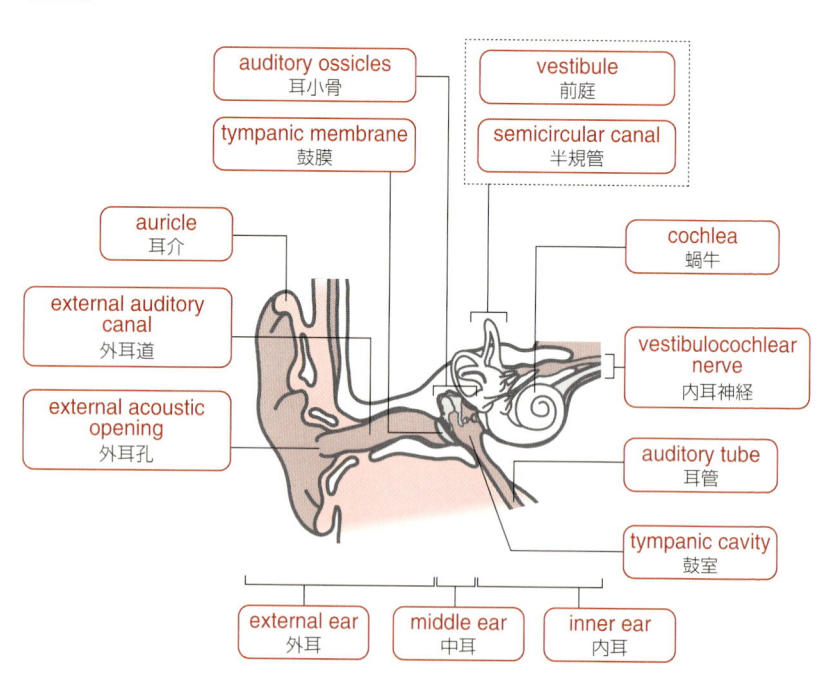

4 耳
Ear
【íər】

解剖図

- auditory ossicles 耳小骨
- tympanic membrane 鼓膜
- vestibule 前庭
- semicircular canal 半規管
- auricle 耳介
- cochlea 蝸牛
- external auditory canal 外耳道
- vestibulocochlear nerve 内耳神経
- external acoustic opening 外耳孔
- auditory tube 耳管
- tympanic cavity 鼓室
- external ear 外耳
- middle ear 中耳
- inner ear 内耳

症候		定義

☐ 093
conductive hearing loss
【kəndʌ́ktiv híəriŋ lɔ́ːs】

伝音難聴

A reduction in the ability to perceive sound due to a <u>lesion</u> in the <u>external auditory canal</u> or the <u>middle ear</u>.
<u>外耳道</u>または<u>中耳</u>の<u>病変</u>による音を知覚する能力の低下.

☐ 094
sensorineural hearing loss
【sènsərin(j)ú(ə)rəl híəriŋ lɔ́ːs】

感音難聴

<u>Hearing loss</u> due to a <u>lesion</u> in the <u>vestibulocochlear nerve</u> or the <u>inner ear</u>.
<u>内耳神経</u>または<u>内耳</u>の<u>病変</u>による<u>難聴</u>.

☐ 095
tinnitus
【tináitəs】

耳鳴り

Perception of a sound in the absence of an environmental <u>acoustic stimulus</u>.
外環境の<u>音刺激</u>が存在しない状態で音を知覚すること.

☐ 096
otalgia[*1]
【outǽldʒiə】

耳痛

Pain in the ear that can be otogenic [*2] or referred from other areas.
耳原性または他の部位から投射された耳の痛み.

> *1 otalgia 名耳痛＝ earache
> *2 otogenic 形耳原性の

☐ 097
otorrhea
【òutəríːə】

耳漏

A <u>discharge</u> from the ear, usually associated with <u>inflammation</u> of the <u>external ear</u> or <u>middle ear</u>.
耳からの<u>排出物</u>. 通常は<u>外耳</u>または<u>中耳</u>の<u>炎症</u>と関連する.

症候		定義

□ **098**

cerumen^{*1}　　耳垢

【sirúːmən】

A waxy substance secreted ^{*2} by the **ceruminous glands** of the **external auditory canal**.
外耳道の**耳道腺**により分泌されたろう様の物質.

* 1　cerumen 名 耳垢＝ earwax
* 2　secrete 動 分泌する

Chapter 4 Vocabulary

Chapter4 に収載している医学関連用語の一覧です

英語	日本語
acoustic stimulus	音刺激
ceruminous gland	耳道腺
discharge	排出物
external auditory canal	外耳道
external ear	外耳
hearing loss	難聴

英語	日本語
inflammation	炎症
inner ear	内耳
lesion	病変
middle ear	中耳
vestibulocochlear nerve	内耳神経

Chapter 5

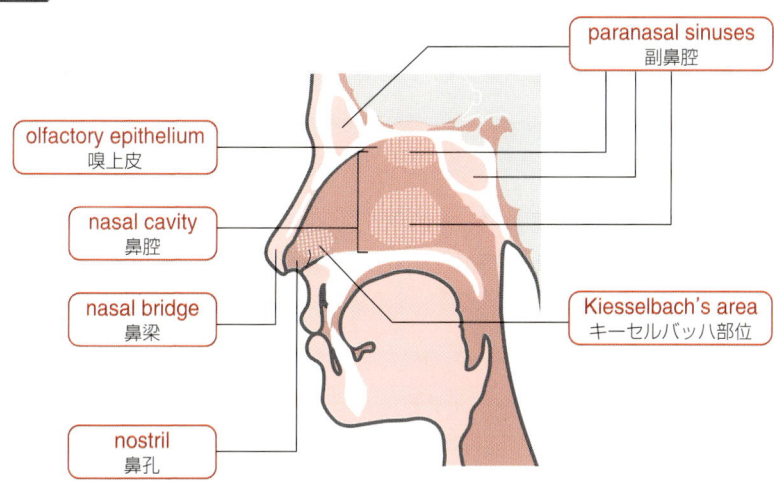

鼻
Nose
【nóuz】

解剖図

- paranasal sinuses 副鼻腔
- olfactory epithelium 嗅上皮
- nasal cavity 鼻腔
- nasal bridge 鼻梁
- Kiesselbach's area キーセルバッハ部位
- nostril 鼻孔

症候		定義

☐ 099
parosmia　　嗅覚錯誤
【pərázmiə】

A distortion of the **sense of smell**, often resulting in subjective perception of nonexistent odors.

嗅覚の変調．しばしば存在しないにおいを主観的に知覚する．

☐ 100
saddle nose　　鞍鼻
[sǽdl nóuz]

A prominent **depression** of the nose due to the collapse of the **nasal bridge**.

鼻梁の崩壊による鼻の顕著な**陥没**．

☐ 101
nasal obstruction　　鼻閉
[néizəl əbstrʌ́kʃən]

Narrowing of the **airway**[*1] in the **nasal cavity**.

鼻腔内の**気道**が狭くなること．

*1　airway 名 気道＝ respiratory tract

☐ 102
rhinorrhea　　鼻漏
[ràinərí:ə]

Excessive **secretion** of **nasal mucus**.

鼻粘液の過剰な**分泌**．

☐ 103
sneeze　　くしゃみ
[sní:z]

A spasmodic[*1] **contraction** of expiratory[*2] **muscles** caused by **irritation** of the **nasal mucous membrane**.

鼻粘膜の**刺激**に起因する**呼息筋**の痙攣性**収縮**．

*1　spasmodic 形 痙攣性の ← spasm 名 痙攣
*2　expiratory 形 呼息の，呼気の ← expiration 名 呼息，呼気

5 鼻

症候		定義

□ 104
epistaxis *1
【èpəstǽksis】

鼻出血

Hemorrhage from the nose, usually due to rupture of small vessels in **Kiesselbach's area**.

鼻からの<u>出血</u>．通常はキーセルバッハ部位の小血管が破れることに起因する．

*1 epistaxis 名 鼻出血＝nosebleed

□ 105
nasal polyp
【néizəl pálip】

鼻ポリープ

A **mass of tissue** abnormally projecting out from the **mucous membranes** of the nose and **paranasal sinuses**.

鼻や<u>副鼻腔</u>の<u>粘膜</u>から異常に突出している<u>組織塊</u>．

Chapter 5 Vocabulary

Chapter5に収載している医学関連用語の一覧です

英語	日本語	英語	日本語
airway	気道	mucous membrane	粘膜
contraction	収縮	nasal bridge	鼻梁
depression	陥没	nasal cavity	鼻腔
expiratory muscle	呼息筋	nasal mucous membrane	鼻粘膜
hemorrhage	出血	nasal mucus	鼻粘液
irritation	刺激	paranasal sinus	副鼻腔
Kiesselbach's area	キーセルバッハ部位	secretion	分泌
mass of tissue	組織塊	sense of smell	嗅覚

Chapter

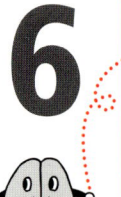

6

呼吸器系

Respiratory System

【réspərətɔ̀:ri sístəm】

解剖図

- nasal cavity 鼻腔
- soft palate 軟口蓋
- nostril 鼻孔
- pharynx 咽頭
- oral cavity 口腔
- larynx 喉頭
- upper respiratory tract 上気道
- vocal cords 声帯
- trachea 気管
- lower respiratory tract 下気道
- bronchi 気管支
- lobar bronchi 葉気管支
- lung 肺
- bronchiole 細気管支
- diaphragm 横隔膜
- alveoli 肺胞

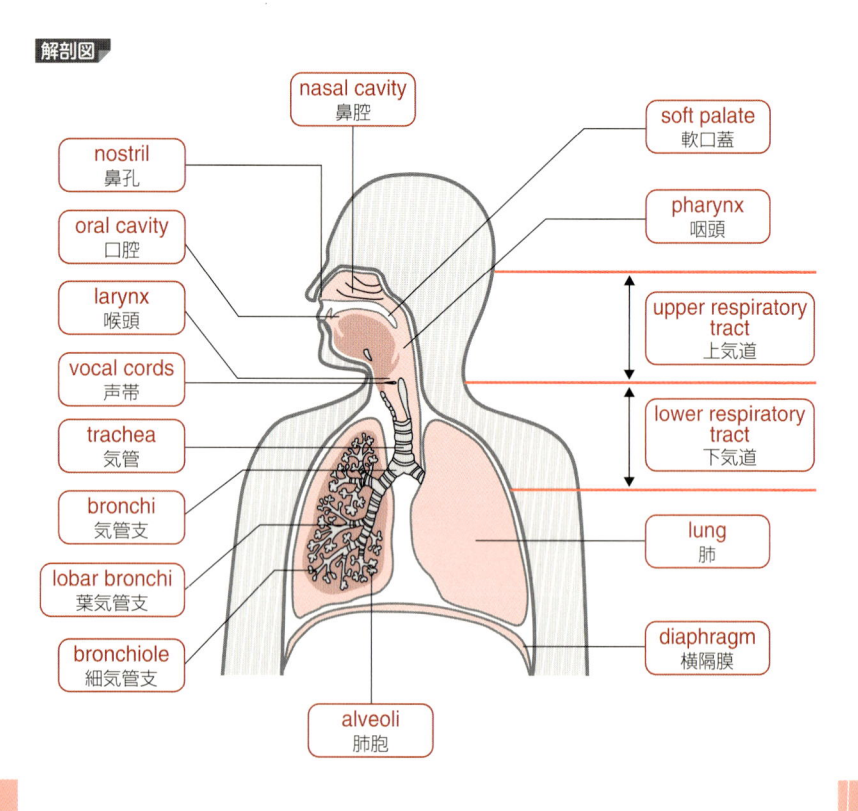

6 呼吸器系

症候 | **定義**

□ 106
snore
【snɔ́:r】

いびき

A rough inspiratory [*1] noise produced by vibration of the <u>soft palate</u> during sleep.

睡眠中に**軟口蓋**の振動により生じる粗い吸息性雑音.

- [*1] inspiratory 形 吸息の, 吸気の ← inspiration 名 吸息, 吸気

□ 107
cough
【kɔ́:f】

咳

A sudden expulsion of air from the <u>lungs</u> caused by <u>irritation</u> of the <u>mucous membranes</u> lining [*1] the <u>trachea</u> and <u>bronchi</u> [*2].

気管および**気管支**の内側を被う**粘膜**の**刺激**に起因する**肺**からの空気の突然の排出.

- [*1] line 動 内側を被う
- [*2] bronchi 名 気管支(複数形;単数形は bronchus)

□ 108
sputum
【spjú:təm】

痰

<u>Mucus</u> or <u>purulent matter</u> expectorated [*1] in diseases of the <u>respiratory tract</u>.

気道の疾患において喀出された**粘液**または**膿性物質**.

- [*1] expectorate 動 喀出する ➡ expectoration 名 喀出

□ 109
hemoptysis
【himáptəsis】

喀血

<u>Expectoration</u> of blood from the <u>respiratory tract</u>.

気道からの血液の**喀出**.

症候		定義

☐ 110
hoarseness 　嗄声
【hɔ́ːrsnəs】

Abnormally rough voice caused by <u>inflammation</u> or injury of the <u>vocal cords</u>.

<u>声帯</u>の<u>炎症</u>または損傷に起因する異常に粗い声．

☐ 111
pleural effusion 　胸水
【plúrəl ifjúːʒən】

An excessive accumulation of fluid within the <u>pleural cavity</u>, usually classified as <u>transudate</u> or <u>exudate</u>.

<u>胸膜腔</u>における液体の過剰な貯留．通常，<u>漏出液</u>と<u>滲出液</u>に分類される．

☐ 112
Kussmaul respiration 　クスマウル呼吸
【kúːsmɔːl rèspəréiʃən】

Deep and rapid <u>respiration</u> characteristic of <u>metabolic acidosis</u>, particularly <u>diabetic</u>[*1] <u>ketoacidosis</u>.

<u>代謝性アシドーシス</u>，特に<u>糖尿病性ケトアシドーシス</u>に特徴的な深く速い<u>呼吸</u>．

*1 diabetic 形 糖尿病(性)の ← diabetes 名 糖尿病

☐ 113
Cheyne-Stokes respiration 　チェーン・ストークス呼吸
【tʃéin- stóuks rèspəréiʃən】

<u>Periodic respiration</u> with a gradual increase in depth followed by a gradual decrease resulting in <u>apnea</u>.

深さが漸増，漸減した後に<u>無呼吸</u>となる<u>周期性呼吸</u>．

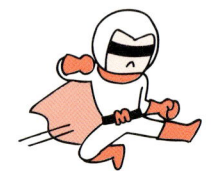

6 呼吸器系

症候 | **定義**

□ 114
Biot respiration ビオー呼吸
[bíːɔ rèspəréiʃən]

An abnormal breathing pattern with continually variable rate and depth of breathing followed by **apnea**.

呼吸の速さや深さが連続して変化した後に<u>無呼吸</u>となる異常な呼吸パターン．

□ 115
orthopnea 起坐呼吸
[ɔːrθápniə]

<u>Difficulty in breathing</u> brought on or aggravated[*1] by lying flat.

水平に横たわることにより発生または悪化する<u>呼吸困難</u>．

*1 aggravate 動 悪化させる

□ 116
prolonged expiration 呼気延長
[proulɔ́ːŋd èkspəréiʃən]

Abnormally long duration of <u>expiration</u> due to difficulty in expelling air from the <u>lungs</u>.

<u>肺</u>からの空気排出の困難による<u>呼気</u>の異常に長い継続．

□ 117
bronchospasm 気管支痙攣
[bráŋkouspæzm]

<u>Contraction</u> of the <u>smooth muscle</u> in the walls of the <u>bronchi</u> and <u>bronchioles</u>, causing <u>stenosis</u> of the <u>lumen</u>.

<u>気管支</u>および<u>細気管支</u>壁の<u>平滑筋</u>の<u>収縮</u>で，<u>管腔</u>の<u>狭窄</u>を引き起こす．

症候		定義

118
coarse crackle 水泡音
【kɔ́ːrs krǽkl】

A discontinuous low-pitched sound heard mostly during **inspiration**, caused by the bursting of air bubbles flowing through **secretions** in the **airway**.

主に**吸気**時に聴かれる非連続性の低音で，**気道**の**分泌物**中を流れる気泡が破裂することにより生じる．

119
fine crackle 捻髪音
【fáin krǽkl】

A discontinuous high-pitched sound heard mostly during **inspiration**, caused by the opening of collapsed **distal**[*1] **airways** and **alveoli**[*2].

主に**吸気**時に聴かれる非連続性の高音で，閉塞した**末梢気道**や**肺胞**が開くことにより生じる．

*1 distal 形 末梢の，遠位の ⟷ proximal 形 近位の
*2 alveoli 名 肺胞（複数形；単数形は alveolus）

120
wheeze 喘鳴
【wiːz】

A continuous high-pitched sound heard mostly during **expiration**, caused by **airway obstruction** from **swelling**, **secretions**, or **spasm**.

主に**呼気**時に聴かれる連続性の高音で，**腫れ**，**分泌物**，または**痙攣**による**気道閉塞**に起因する．

121
rhonchus いびき様音
【rɑ́ŋkəs】

A continuous low-pitched sound with a snoring quality usually associated with **secretions** in large **airways**.

主に太い**気道**内の**分泌物**に関連するいびき様の連続性の低音．

6 呼吸器系

| 症 候 | | 定 義 |

☐ 122
decreased breath sound
【dikríːst bréθ sáund】

呼吸音減弱

Reduced transmission of **breath sound** across the **chest wall** due to decreased flow of air through the **airway**.
気道内の空気の流れの減少により**胸壁**の外への**呼吸音**の伝達が低下すること.

☐ 123
pleural rub
【plúərəl rʌ́b】

胸膜摩擦音

Friction sound caused by rubbing of the roughened surfaces of the **costal**[*1] **pleura** and the **pulmonary**[*2] **pleura**.
肋骨胸膜と**肺胸膜**の荒れた表面が擦れ合うことにより生じる**摩擦音**.

*1 costal 形 肋骨の ← costa 名 肋骨
*2 pulmonary 形 肺の

☐ 124
egophony
【iːgáfəni】

山羊声

Voice sounds resembling the bleating of a goat caused by compressed **lung tissue** due to **pleural effusion**.
胸水により圧迫された**肺組織**に起因する山羊の鳴き声に似た声音.

☐ 125
vocal fremitus
【vóukəl frémitəs】

声音震盪

Vibration in the **chest wall** produced by the spoken voice that is felt on **palpation**.
話し声により生じ,**触診**で感じられる**胸壁**内の振動.

症 候		定 義

☐ 126

dyspnea 呼吸困難
【dispníːə】

A subjective sensation of <u>shortness of breath</u> usually associated with cardiopulmonary [*1] disease.

主に心肺の疾患に関連する主観的な<u>息切れ</u>の感覚．

* [1] cardiopulmonary 形 心肺の

☐ 127

apnea 無呼吸
【ǽpniə】

Transient cessation of <u>respiration</u>, often resulting in <u>hypoxemia</u>.

<u>呼吸</u>の一時的な停止．しばしば<u>低酸素血症</u>を生じる．

☐ 128

tachypnea 頻呼吸
【tækipníːə】

Increase in <u>respiratory rate</u> usually associated with <u>heart failure</u>, <u>pulmonary embolism</u>, or <u>pneumonia</u>.

主に<u>心不全</u>，<u>肺塞栓症</u>，<u>肺炎</u>に関連する<u>呼吸数</u>の増加．

☐ 129

hyperventilation 過換気
【hàipərvèntəléiʃən】

Increased <u>alveolar</u>[*1] <u>ventilation</u> relative to metabolic <u>carbon dioxide</u> production, leading to a loss of <u>carbon dioxide</u> from the blood.

代謝による<u>二酸化炭素</u>産生に比較して<u>肺胞換気</u>が亢進している状態で，血液中の<u>二酸化炭素</u>の減少を引き起こす．

* [1] alveolar 形 肺胞の ← alveolus 名 肺胞

6 呼吸器系

Chapter6 Vocabulary

Chapter6に収載している医学関連用語の一覧です

英語	日本語
airway	気道
airway obstruction	気道閉塞
alveolar ventilation	肺胞換気
alveoli(alveolus)	肺胞
apnea	無呼吸
breath sound	呼吸音
bronchi(bronchus)	気管支
bronchiole	細気管支
carbon dioxide	二酸化炭素
chest wall	胸壁
contraction	収縮
costal pleura	肋骨胸膜
diabetic ketoacidosis	糖尿病性ケトアシドーシス
difficulty in breathing	呼吸困難
distal airway	末梢気道
expectoration	喀出
expiration	呼気
exudate	滲出液
friction sound	摩擦音
heart failure	心不全
hypoxemia	低酸素血症
inflammation	炎症
inspiration	吸気
irritation	刺激
lumen	管腔
lung tissue	肺組織

英語	日本語
lung	肺
metabolic acidosis	代謝性アシドーシス
mucous membrane	粘膜
mucus	粘液
palpation	触診
periodic respiration	周期性呼吸
pleural cavity	胸膜腔
pleural effusion	胸水
pneumonia	肺炎
pulmonary embolism	肺塞栓症
pulmonary pleura	肺胸膜
purulent matter	膿性物質
respiration	呼吸
respiratory rate	呼吸数
respiratory tract	気道
secretion	分泌物
shortness of breath	息切れ
smooth muscle	平滑筋
soft palate	軟口蓋
spasm	痙攣
stenosis	狭窄
swelling	腫れ
trachea	気管
transudate	漏出液
vocal cord	声帯

Chapter

7

循環器系
Circulatory System
【sə́:rkjulətɔ̀:ri sístəm】

解剖図

- aortic arch 大動脈弓
- superior vena cava 上大静脈
- ascending aorta 上行大動脈
- right atrium 右心房
- tricuspid valve 三尖弁 (atrioventricular valve)(房室弁)
- right ventricle 右心室
- inferior vena cava 下大静脈
- arterial ligament 動脈管索
- pulmonary artery 肺動脈
- aortic valve 大動脈弁 (semilunar valve)(半月弁)
- left atrium 左心房
- mitral valve 僧帽弁 (atrioventricular valve)(房室弁)
- left ventricle 左心室
- interventricular septum 心室中隔

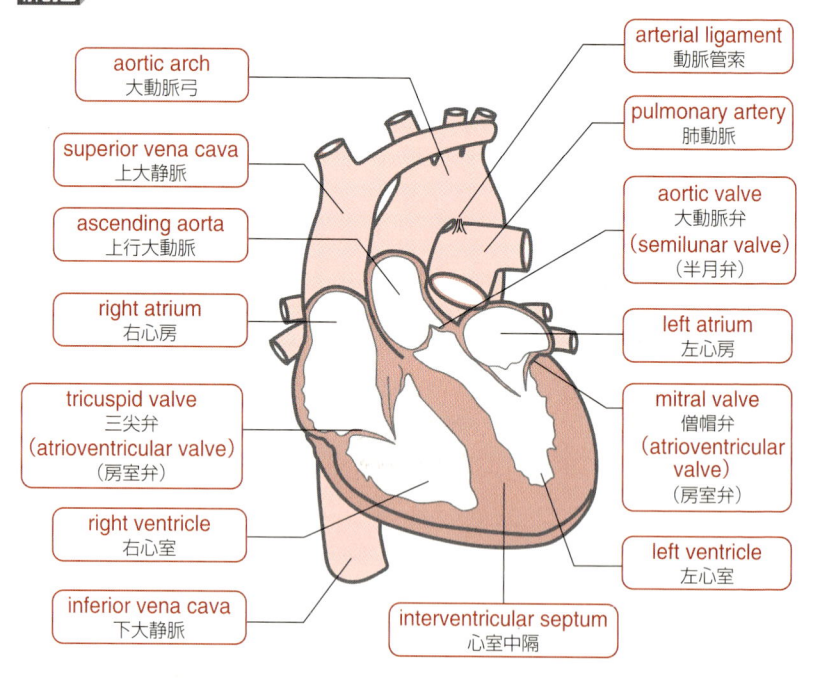

その症候、英語で言えますか？

7 循環器系

症候 / 定義

130

third heart sound Ⅲ音
【θə́:rd hɑ́:rt sáund】

An **extra heart sound** in early **diastole** associated with rapid **ventricular**[*1] **filling**.
急速な心室充満に関連する拡張期早期の過剰心音.

*1 ventricular 形 心室の ← ventricle 名 心室

131

fourth heart sound Ⅳ音
【fɔ́:rθ hɑ́:rt sáund】

An **extra heart sound** in late **diastole** associated with **atrial**[*1] **systole**.
心房収縮に関連する拡張期末期の過剰心音.

*1 atrial 形 心房の ← atrium 名 心房

132

opening snap 開放音
【óupəniŋ snǽp】

A diastolic[*1] sound caused by the opening of a stenotic[*2] **atrioventricular valve**.
狭窄した房室弁の開放により生じる拡張期の音.

*1 diastolic 形 拡張期の ← diastole 名 拡張期
*2 stenotic 形 狭窄した ← stenosis 名 狭窄

133

midsystolic click 収縮中期クリック
【míd-sistálik klík】

A high-pitched sound produced in the middle of **systole** by **mitral valve prolapse**.
僧帽弁逸脱により収縮期の中期に生じる高音.

症候		定義

☐ 134

gallop rhythm 　奔馬調律　A disordered rhythm of the heart characterized by the presence of the third or fourth heart sound in addition to the first and second sounds.
【gǽləp ríðm】

　　　　　Ⅰ音，Ⅱ音に加えⅢ音またはⅣ音の存在を特徴とする心臓の乱れたリズム．

☐ 135

innocent murmur 　無害性雑音　A **cardiac** *¹ **murmur** caused by minor turbulence in **blood flow** in a healthy heart.
【ínəsənt mə́ːrmər】

　　　　　健康な心臓における<u>血流</u>の軽度の乱れに起因する<u>心雑音</u>．

＊1 cardiac 形 心臓の

☐ 136

systolic ejection murmur 　収縮期駆出性雑音　A <u>murmur</u> caused by the <u>ejection</u> of blood into the <u>aorta</u> or <u>pulmonary artery</u>.
【sistálik idʒékʃən mə́ːrmər】

　　　　　<u>大動脈</u>または<u>肺動脈</u>への血液の<u>駆出</u>に起因する<u>雑音</u>．

☐ 137

pansystolic murmur 　汎収縮期雑音　A <u>murmur</u> occupying the entire <u>systole</u>, caused by backward flow across the <u>atrioventricular valves</u>.
【pæn-sistálik mə́ːrmər】

　　　　　<u>収縮期</u>全体にわたる<u>雑音</u>で，<u>房室弁</u>での逆流に起因する．

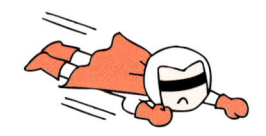

7 循環器系

症候		定義

☐ **138**
diastolic regurgitant murmur
【dàiəstɑ́lik rigə́ːrdʒətənt mə́ːrmər】

拡張期逆流性雑音

A <u>murmur</u> accompanying backward flow across <u>semilunar valves</u>.
<u>半月弁</u>での逆流に伴う<u>雑音</u>.

☐ **139**
middiastolic murmur
【míd-dàiəstɑ́lik mə́ːrmər】

拡張中期雑音

A <u>murmur</u> caused by turbulent flow across the <u>atrioventricular valves</u>.
<u>房室弁</u>での乱流に起因する<u>雑音</u>.

☐ **140**
continuous murmur
【kəntínjuəs mə́ːrmər】

連続性雑音

A <u>murmur</u> heard without interruption throughout <u>systole</u> and into <u>diastole</u>.
<u>収縮期</u>から<u>拡張期</u>にかけて中断なく聴かれる<u>雑音</u>.

☐ **141**
pericardial friction rub
【pèrəkɑ́ːrdiəl fríkʃən rʌ́b】

心膜摩擦音

A grating sound caused by rubbing of the inflamed pericardial[*1] surfaces.
炎症を起こした心膜表面が擦れ合うことにより生じる軋み音.

＊1 pericardial 形 心膜の ← pericardium 名 心膜

症候		定義

142
venous hum
【víːnəs hʌm】

静脈こま音

A continuous low-pitched sound caused by turbulent flow in the <u>jugular veins</u>.
<u>頸静脈</u>内の乱流に起因する連続性の低音.

143
carotid bruit
【kərátid brúːt】

頸動脈雑音

A <u>systolic murmur</u> caused by turbulent flow in the <u>carotid arteries</u> [*1].
<u>頸動脈</u>内の乱流に起因する<u>収縮期雑音</u>.

[*1] carotid artery 名頸動脈（単に carotid ともいう）

144
arrhythmia
【əríðmiə】

不整脈

An irregularity in the rate or rhythm of the <u>heartbeat</u>.
<u>心拍</u>の速さまたはリズムの不規則性.

145
tachycardia
【tækikáːrdiə】

頻脈

A rapid <u>heartbeat</u>, usually applied to a rate over 100 beats per minute.
速い<u>心拍</u>. 通常は毎分100拍以上をいう.

146
bradycardia
【brædikáːrdiə】

徐脈

A slow <u>heartbeat</u>, usually applied to a rate under 60 beats per minute.
遅い<u>心拍</u>. 通常は毎分60拍以下をいう.

147
pulsus celer
【pʌ́lsəs síːlər】

速脈

A <u>pulse</u> swift to rise and fall.
急速に上昇し下降する<u>脈拍</u>.

7 循環器系

症候 | **定義**

□ **148**

pulsus tardus 遅脈
【pʌ́lsəs tάːrdʌs】

A **pulse** with an abnormally gradual upstroke.
異常にゆるやかな立ち上がりを示す**脈拍**.

□ **149**

alternating pulse *¹ 交互脈
【ɔ́ːltərnèitiŋ pʌ́ls】

A **pulse** with alternating strong and weak beats.
強弱の拍動が交互に現われる**脈拍**.

* 1 alternating pulse 名 交互脈＝pulsus alternans

□ **150**

paradoxical pulse *¹ 奇脈
【pærədάksikəl pʌ́ls】

An exaggerated drop in **systolic pressure** during **inspiration**.
吸気時における**収縮期圧**の極端な下降.

* 1 paradoxical pulse 名 奇脈＝pulsus paradoxus

□ **151**

palpitation 動悸
【pælpətéiʃən】

A subjective sensation of an irregular or abnormal **heartbeat**.
不規則または異常な**心拍**の主観的な感覚.

□ **152**

cardiac arrest 心停止
【kάːrdiæk ərést】

Complete cessation of electrical and mechanical activities of the heart.
心臓の電気的および機械的活動の完全な停止.

症候		定義

153
hypertension
【haipərténʃən】

高血圧

Abnormally high <u>blood pressure</u>, usually applied to a <u>systolic blood pressure</u> above 140 mmHg or a <u>diastolic blood pressure</u> above 90 mmHg.

異常に高い<u>血圧</u>．通常は<u>収縮期血圧</u>が140 mmHg以上，または<u>拡張期血圧</u>が90 mmHg以上をいう．

154
hypotension
【haipouténʃən】

低血圧

Abnormally low <u>blood pressure</u>, usually applied to a <u>systolic blood pressure</u> under 100 mmHg.

異常に低い<u>血圧</u>．通常は<u>収縮期血圧</u>が100 mmHg以下をいう．

155
intermittent claudication
【intərmítnt klɔ̀:dəkéiʃən】

間欠性跛行

Pain and <u>cramps</u> in the <u>calf</u> muscles due to <u>ischemia</u> that are brought on by walking.

<u>虚血</u>によるふくらはぎ筋肉の痛みおよび<u>痙攣</u>で，歩行により生じる．

156
syncope
【síŋkəpi:】

失神

Loss of <u>consciousness</u> caused by diminished cerebral*1 <u>blood flow</u>.

大脳の<u>血流</u>低下に起因する<u>意識</u>の喪失．

*1 cerebral 形 大脳の ← cerebrum 名 大脳

157
Adams-Stokes syndrome
【ǽdəmz-stóuks síndroum】

アダムズ・ストークス症候群

Slow or absent <u>pulse</u> as a result of <u>atrioventricular block</u>, causing <u>syncope</u> with or without <u>convulsions</u>.

<u>房室ブロック</u>に起因する<u>脈拍</u>の低下または消失．<u>失神</u>を引き起こし，<u>けいれん</u>を伴うこともある．

7 循環器系

症候 | **定義**

☐ 158
cyanosis
【sàiənóusis】

チアノーゼ

A bluish or purplish <u>discoloration</u> of the skin and <u>mucous membranes</u> due to deficient <u>oxygenation</u> of the blood.

血液の<u>酸素化</u>の不足による皮膚および<u>粘膜</u>の青色または紫色の<u>変色</u>.

☐ 159
hypoxemia
【hàipaksí:miə】

低酸素血症

Decreased <u>oxygen partial pressure</u> in arterial[*1] blood.

<u>動脈血</u>中の<u>酸素分圧</u>の低下.

＊1 arterial 形動脈の ← artery 名動脈

☐ 160
varicose veins
【værəkòus veinz】

拡張蛇行
静脈

Abnormal <u>dilation</u> and tortuosity of <u>superficial veins</u>, usually seen in the legs.

<u>表在静脈</u>の異常な<u>拡張</u>および蛇行. 通常は下肢にみられる.

Chapter 7 Vocabulary

Chapter7に収載している医学関連用語の一覧です

英語	日本語	英語	日本語
aorta	大動脈	blood pressure	血圧
arterial blood	動脈血	calf	ふくらはぎ
atrial systole	心房収縮	cardiac murmur	心雑音
atrioventricular block	房室ブロック	carotid artery	頸動脈
atrioventricular valve	房室弁	consciousness	意識
blood flow	血流	convulsion	けいれん

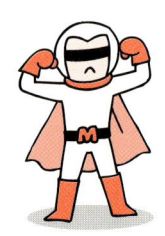

英語	日本語
cramp	痙攣
diastole	拡張期
diastolic blood pressure	拡張期血圧
dilation	拡張
discoloration	変色
ejection	駆出
extra heart sound	過剰心音
heartbeat	心拍
inspiration	吸気
ischemia	虚血
jugular vein	頸静脈
mitral valve prolapse	僧帽弁逸脱
mucous membrane	粘膜
murmur	雑音
oxygen partial pressure	酸素分圧
oxygenation	酸素化
pulmonary artery	肺動脈
pulse	脈拍
semilunar valve	半月弁
superficial vein	表在静脈
syncope	失神
systole	収縮期
systolic blood pressure	収縮期血圧
systolic murmur	収縮期雑音
systolic pressure	収縮期圧
ventricular filling	心室充満

Chapter 8

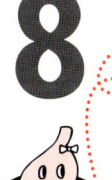

消化器系
Digestive System
【daidʒéstiv sístəm】

解剖図

- nasal cavity / 鼻腔
- oral cavity / 口腔
- larynx / 喉頭
- liver / 肝臓
- gallbladder / 胆嚢
- duodenum / 十二指腸
- ascending colon / 上行結腸
- ileum / 回腸
- cecum / 盲腸
- appendix / 虫垂
- rectum / 直腸
- pharynx / 咽頭
- esophagus / 食道
- stomach / 胃
- spleen / 脾臓
- pancreas / 膵臓
- transverse colon / 横行結腸
- jejunum / 空腸
- descending colon / 下行結腸
- sigmoid colon / S状結腸
- anus / 肛門

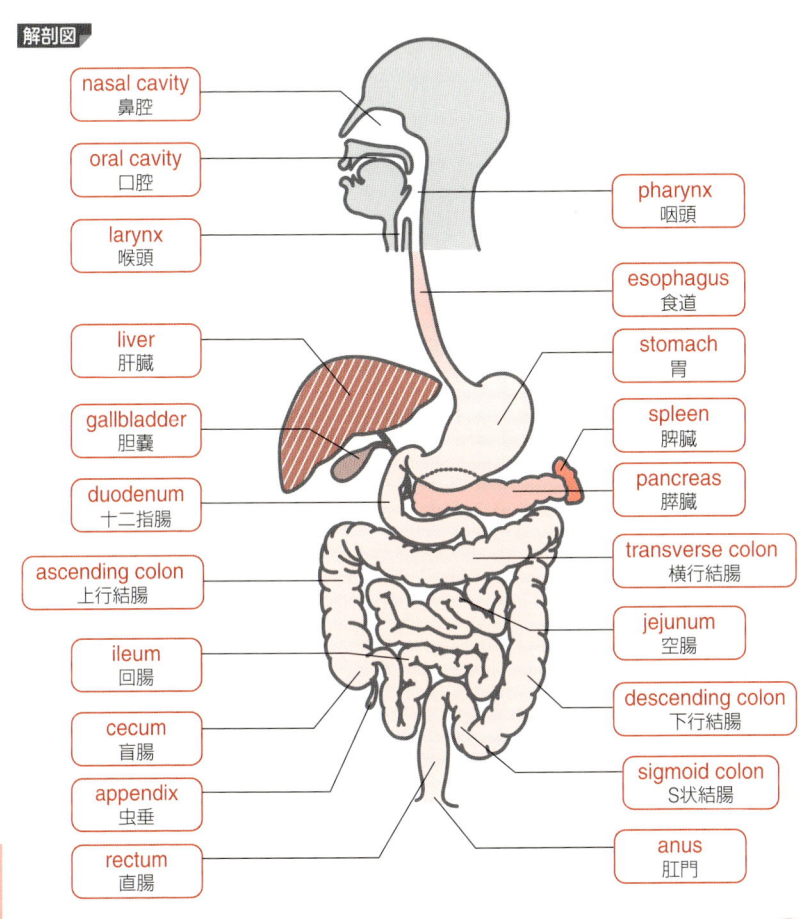

症候		定義

☐ 161
dysgeusia 味覚異常 Unpleasant alteration of the <u>sense of taste</u> or decrease in taste <u>sensitivity</u>.
【disgjúːʒiə】

味覚の不快な変化または味の**感受性**の低下．

☐ 162
hyposalivation 唾液分泌不全 An abnormal reduction in the <u>secretion</u> of <u>saliva</u>.
【háipousæləvéiʃən】

唾液の**分泌**の異常な低下．

☐ 163
tongue coating 舌苔 A moss-like <u>deposit</u> over the <u>tongue</u> surface including desquamated*1 <u>epithelium</u>, <u>leukocytes</u>,
【tʌ́ŋ kóutiŋ】 food debris, and <u>bacteria</u>*2.

<u>舌</u>表面の苔様の**沈着物**で，剥離した<u>上皮</u>，<u>白血球</u>，食物かす，**細菌**を含む．

> *1 desquamated 形 剥離した ➡ desquamation 名 剥離，落屑
> *2 bacteria 名 細菌（複数形；単数形は bacterium）

☐ 164
strawberry イチゴ舌 A <u>tongue</u> with whitish coat where enlarged <u>lingual</u>
tongue <u>papillae</u>*1 project as red points.
【strɔ́ːbèri tʌ́ŋ】

白い舌苔から肥大した**舌乳頭**が赤い点状に突出している<u>舌</u>．

> *1 lingual papillae 名 舌乳頭（複数形；通常は複数形を使用する）

その症候，英語で言えますか？

8 消化器系

症候 / 定義

□ 165

macroglossia 巨大舌
【mækrəglásiə】

Enlargement of the tongue due to abnormal tissue growth or accumulation of material.

異常な組織増殖または物質の蓄積による舌の肥大.

□ 166

dental caries う歯
【déntl kǽriz】

Destruction of calcified[*1] tissue of the tooth by organic acids produced by bacteria in the oral cavity.

口腔内の細菌により産生された有機酸による歯の石灰化組織の破壊.

*1 calcified 形 石灰化した ➡ calcification 名 石灰化

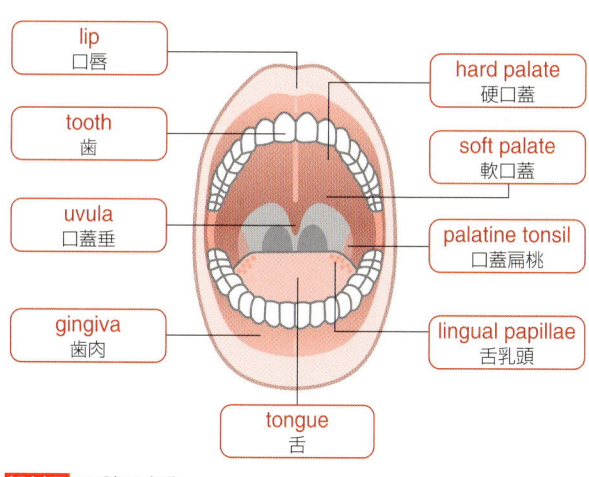

- lip 口唇
- tooth 歯
- uvula 口蓋垂
- gingiva 歯肉
- tongue 舌
- hard palate 硬口蓋
- soft palate 軟口蓋
- palatine tonsil 口蓋扁桃
- lingual papillae 舌乳頭

解剖図 口腔の名称

症候		定義

☐ 167
halitosis 口臭
【hǽlətóusis】

A foul odor from the mouth usually due to **volatile**[*1] **sulfur**[*2] **compounds** produced by **oral bacteria**.

口からの悪臭で，通常は<u>口内細菌</u>により産生された<u>揮発性硫化化合物</u>による．

- *1 volatile 形 揮発性の
- *2 sulfur 名 硫黄

☐ 168
fetor hepaticus 肝性口臭
【fí:tər hipǽtikʌs】

A peculiar odor to the breath caused by **volatile aromatic**[*1] **substances** in the blood and **urine** due to defective hepatic[*2] **metabolism**.

肝臓の<u>代謝</u>不全に起因する血液および<u>尿</u>中の<u>揮発性芳香族物質</u>により生じる息の独特なにおい．

- *1 aromatic 形 芳香族の
- *2 hepatic 形 肝臓の

☐ 169
trismus 開口障害
【trízməs】

Persistent **contraction** of the **masseter muscles**, typically as an initial **symptom** of **tetanus**.

<u>咬筋</u>の持続的な<u>収縮</u>で，<u>破傷風</u>の典型的な初期症状．

☐ 170
dysmasesis 咀嚼障害
【dismə́sí:sis】

Difficulty in **mastication** due to **malocclusion** or **dysfunction** of the **masticatory muscles**.

<u>不正咬合</u>または<u>咀嚼筋</u>の<u>機能不全</u>による<u>咀嚼</u>の困難．

8 消化器系

症候		定義

□ 171
dysphagia
【dìsféidʒiə】

嚥下障害

Difficulty in **swallowing** due to a **neuromuscular disorder**, **spasm**, or **esophageal**[*1] **obstruction**.
神経筋障害，痙攣，または食道閉塞による嚥下の困難．

[*1] esophageal 形 食道の ← esophagus 名 食道

□ 172
hiccup
【híkʌp】

しゃっくり

A **spasm** of the **diaphragm** accompanied by a rapid closure of the **glottis**.
声門の急速な閉鎖を伴う横隔膜の痙攣．

□ 173
pyrosis[*1]
【pairóusis】

胸やけ

Substernal[*2] pain or **burning sensation** caused by **regurgitation** of **gastric juice** into the **esophagus**.
食道への胃液の逆流に起因する胸骨下の痛みまたは灼熱感．

[*1] pyrosis 名 胸やけ = heartburn
[*2] substernal 形 胸骨下の ← sternum 名 胸骨

□ 174
eructation
【irʌktéiʃən】

おくび

Emission of gas from the **stomach** through the mouth.
口を通じて胃からガスを放出すること．

□ 175
flatus
【fléitəs】

放屁

Emission of gas from the **gastrointestinal tract** through the **anus**.
肛門を通じて胃腸管からガスを放出すること．

症候		定義

☐ 176
nausea 悪心
[nɔ́:ziə]

An unpleasant sensation in the **stomach** characterized by an urge to vomit*¹.

吐き気を特徴とする胃の不快感.

＊1 vomit 動 嘔吐する

☐ 177
emesis＊¹ 嘔吐
[émǝsis]

A **reflex movement** in which the contents of the **stomach** are ejected through the mouth.

胃の内容物が口から排出される反射運動.

＊1 emesis 名 嘔吐 ＝ vomiting

☐ 178
visceral pain 内臓痛
[vísǝrǝl péin]

Dull pain due to **spasm**, **obstruction**, or **distention** of any of the **hollow viscera**＊¹.

いずれかの管腔臓器の痙攣，閉塞，または膨張による鈍い痛み.

＊1 viscera 名 内臓（複数形；単数形は viscus）

☐ 179
somatic pain 体性痛
[soumǽtik péin]

Pain in **tissues** such as skin, **mucous membranes**, muscles, and bones that is easier to locate and more intense than **visceral pain**.

皮膚，粘膜，筋肉，骨などの組織における痛みで，内臓痛より場所の特定が容易で痛みも強い.

☐ 180
referred pain 関連痛
[rifə́:rd péin]

Pain perceived in a region separate from its actual origin.

実際の起源から離れた部位で感じられる痛み.

症候		定義

181
muscular defense 筋性防御
【mʌ́skjulər diféns】

A <u>reflex</u> of <u>abdominal muscles</u> to contract upon pressure to the <u>abdomen</u>.
<u>腹部</u>への圧力に対し<u>腹筋</u>が収縮する<u>反射</u>.

182
rebound tenderness[*1] 反跳圧痛
【ribáund téndərnəs】

Pain experienced on sudden release of steadily applied pressure on the <u>abdomen</u>.
<u>腹部</u>に徐々に加えた圧力を急に解放した際に感じられる痛み.

* 1 rebound tenderness 名 反跳圧痛 = Blumberg sign 名 ブルンベルグ徴候

183
caput medusae メズサの頭
【kǽpət midjúːziː】

Dilated <u>paraumbilical veins</u> radiating from the <u>umbilicus</u> across the <u>abdomen</u>.
<u>臍</u>から<u>腹部</u>に放射状に広がる拡張した<u>臍傍静脈</u>.

184
anorexia 食欲不振
【æ̀nəréksiə】

Loss of <u>appetite</u> or <u>aversion</u> to food.
<u>食欲</u>の消失または食物に対する<u>嫌悪</u>.

185
hyperphagia 過食症
【hàipərféidʒiə】

Abnormally increased <u>appetite</u> for and <u>ingestion</u> of food.
異常に亢進した<u>食欲</u>および食物<u>摂取</u>.

症候		定義

186
dyspepsia 消化不良
【dispépsiə】

A disorder of **digestive function** characterized by **epigastric**[*1] **pain**, **heartburn**, or **nausea**.

上腹部痛，胸やけ，悪心を特徴とする消化機能の障害．

> [*1] epigastric 形 上腹部の ← epigastrium 名 上腹部，心窩部

187
malabsorption 吸収不良
【mæləbzɔ́ːrpʃən】

Impaired **absorption** of **nutrients** from the **alimentary canal**.

消化管からの栄養分の吸収における障害．

188
gastric dilatation 胃拡張
【gǽstrik dilətéiʃən】

Enlargement of the **stomach**, usually due to **obstruction** of the **pyloric**[*1] **valve**.

主に幽門弁の閉塞による胃の肥大．

> [*1] pyloric 形 幽門の ← pylorus 名 幽門

189
gastroptosis 胃下垂
【gæstrɑptóusis】

Abnormal downward displacement of the **stomach**.

胃の異常な下方への移動．

190
gastrospasm 胃痙攣
【gǽstrouspæzəm】

Involuntary and often painful **contraction** of the **smooth muscle** of the **gastric wall**.

胃壁の平滑筋のしばしば痛みを伴う不随意な収縮．

8 消化器系

症候 | **定義**

☐ **191**
hyperchlorhydria 胃酸過多
【hàipərklɔ:rháidriə】

Excessive secretion of gastric acid by parietal cells.
壁細胞による胃酸の過剰な分泌.

☐ **192**
hematemesis 吐血
【hì:mətéməsis】

The vomiting of blood, usually due to hemorrhage in the upper gastrointestinal tract.
血液を吐くこと.通常は上部胃腸管の出血による.

☐ **193**
hematochezia 鮮血便
【hemətəkí:ziə】

Passage of stools with bright red blood.
鮮紅色の血液を含む便の排出.

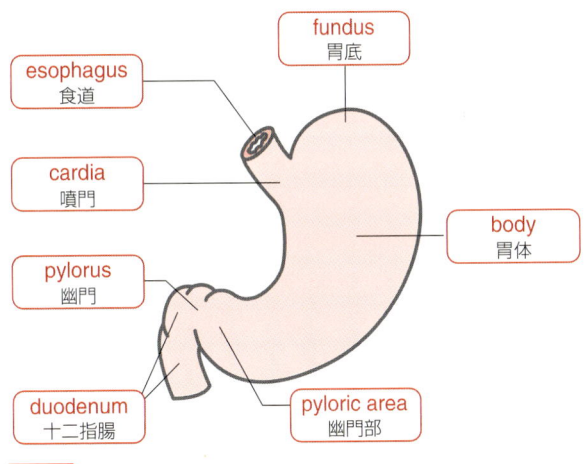

- esophagus 食道
- fundus 胃底
- cardia 噴門
- body 胃体
- pylorus 幽門
- duodenum 十二指腸
- pyloric area 幽門部

解剖図 胃各部の名称

症候		定義

□ 194
melena
【məlíːnə】

黒色便

Passage of black, **tarry stools**.
黒色の**タール様便**の排出.

□ 195
acholic stool
【eikálik stúːl】

無胆汁便

White or abnormally pale **stool** due to lack of **bile pigments**.
胆汁色素の欠如による白色または異常に色が薄い**便**.

□ 196
diarrhea
【dàiəríːə】

下痢

Frequent passage of semisolid or liquid **stools**.
半固体または液状の**便**の頻繁な排出.

□ 197
constipation
【kànstəpéiʃən】

便秘

Difficult or infrequent **bowel movements**.
排便の困難,または頻度低下.

□ 198
tenesmus
【tinézməs】

しぶり

A **spasm** of the **anal**[*1] **sphincter** characterized by a strong desire to defecate[*2], with little or no **stool** passed.
肛門括約筋の**痙攣**で,強い便意を特徴とするが**便**はほとんど排出されない.

> [*1] anal 形 肛門の ← anus 名 肛門
> [*2] defecate 動 排便する

8 消化器系

| 症候 | | 定義 |

199
meteorism　鼓腸
【míːtiərìzm】

Abdominal distention due to swallowed air or intestinal*1 gas from fermentation.

嚥下された空気または発酵による腸内ガスに起因する腹部膨満.

*1 intestinal 形 腸の ← intestine 名 腸

200
borborygmus　腹鳴
【bòːrbərígməs】

A rumbling noise produced by movement of gas or fluid in the alimentary canal.

消化管内のガスや液体の移動によって生じるゴロゴロという音.

201
ascites　腹水
【əsáitiːz】

Accumulation of serous fluid in the peritoneal*1 cavity.

腹膜腔における漿液の貯留.

*1 peritoneal 形 腹膜の ← peritoneum 名 腹膜

202
hepatomegaly　肝腫大
【hepætouméɡəli】

Abnormal enlargement of the liver due to congestion, inflammation, tumor, or metabolic disorders.

うっ血, 炎症, 腫瘍, 代謝性疾患等による肝臓の異常な肥大.

症候			定義

☐ 203
splenomegaly 脾腫
【splenouméɡəli】

Abnormal **enlargement** of the **spleen** due to **infection**, **congestion**, **immune disorders**, or **hematologic**[*1] **disorders**.

感染，うっ血，免疫疾患，血液疾患等による脾臓の異常な肥大．

> *1 hematologic 形 血液の，血液学の ← hematology 名 血液学

☐ 204
abdominal mass 腹部腫瘤
【ӕbdάmənl mӕs】

A localized **swelling**, **induration**, or **enlargement** in the **abdomen**.

腹部に局在する腫れ，硬化，または肥大．

Chapter 8 Vocabulary

Chapter8に収載している医学関連用語の一覧です

英語	日本語	英語	日本語
abdomen	腹部	burning sensation	灼熱感
abdominal distention	腹部膨満	calcified tissue	石灰化組織
abdominal muscle	腹筋	congestion	うっ血
absorption	吸収	contraction	収縮
alimentary canal	消化管	deposit	沈着物
anal sphincter	肛門括約筋	diaphragm	横隔膜
anus	肛門	digestive function	消化機能
appetite	食欲	distention	膨張
aversion	嫌悪	dysfunction	機能不全
bacteria(bacterium)	細菌	enlargement	肥大
bile pigment	胆汁色素	epigastric pain	上腹部痛
bowel movement	排便	epithelium	上皮

8 消化器系

英語	日本語
esophageal obstruction	食道閉塞
esophagus	食道
fermentation	発酵
gastric acid	胃酸
gastric juice	胃液
gastric wall	胃壁
gastrointestinal tract	胃腸管
glottis	声門
heartburn	胸やけ
hematologic disorder	血液疾患
hemorrhage	出血
hollow viscera	管腔臓器
immune disorder	免疫疾患
induration	硬化
infection	感染
inflammation	炎症
ingestion	摂取
intestinal gas	腸内ガス
leukocyte	白血球
lingual papillae	舌乳頭
liver	肝臓
malocclusion	不正咬合
masseter muscle	咬筋
mastication	咀嚼
masticatory muscle	咀嚼筋
metabolic disorder	代謝性疾患
metabolism	代謝
mucous membrane	粘膜
nausea	悪心
neuromuscular disorder	神経筋障害
nutrient	栄養分
obstruction	閉塞
oral bacteria	口内細菌
oral cavity	口腔

英語	日本語
organic acid	有機酸
paraumbilical vein	臍傍静脈
parietal cell	壁細胞
peritoneal cavity	腹膜腔
pyloric valve	幽門弁
reflex	反射
reflex movement	反射運動
regurgitation	逆流
saliva	唾液
secretion	分泌
sense of taste	味覚
sensitivity	感受性
serous fluid	漿液
smooth muscle	平滑筋
spasm	痙攣
spleen	脾臓
stomach	胃
stool	便
swallowing	嚥下
swelling	腫れ
symptom	症状
tarry stool	タール様便
tetanus	破傷風
tissue	組織
tissue growth	組織増殖
tongue	舌
tumor	腫瘍
umbilicus	臍
upper gastrointestinal tract	上部胃腸管
urine	尿
visceral pain	内臓痛
volatile aromatic substance	揮発性芳香族物質
volatile sulfur compound	揮発性硫化化合物

Chapter 9

血液と造血
Blood and Hemopoiesis
【blʌd】 and 【hìːməpɔiíːsis】

模式図

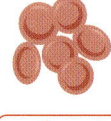

- **erythrocyte** 赤血球
- **platelet** 血小板

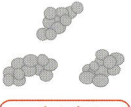

- **basophil** 好塩基球
- **eosinophil** 好酸球
- **neutrophil** 好中球
- **monocyte** 単球
- **lymphocyte** リンパ球

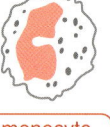

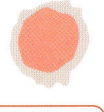

- **granulocyte** 顆粒白血球 (basophil, eosinophil, neutrophil)
- **agranulocyte** 無顆粒白血球 (monocyte, lymphocyte)
- **leukocyte** 白血球

9 血液と造血

| 症 候 | | 定 義 |

□ 205

anemia 貧血
【əníːmiə】

An abnormal decrease in the number of <u>red blood cells</u> *1 or the amount of <u>hemoglobin</u> in the blood.
血中の赤血球の数またはヘモグロビンの量の異常な減少.

＊1 red blood cell 名 赤血球＝erythrocyte

□ 206

polycythemia *1 赤血球増加
【pàlisaiθíːmiə】

An abnormal increase in the number of <u>red blood cells</u>.
赤血球の数の異常な増加.

＊1 polycythemia 名 赤血球増加 ⇔ erythropenia 名 赤血球減少

□ 207

leukocytosis *1 白血球増加
【lùːkousaitóusis】

An abnormal elevation of the <u>white blood cell</u> *2 count.
白血球数の異常な増加.

＊1 leukocytosis 名 白血球増加 ⇔ leukopenia 名 白血球減少
＊2 white blood cell 名 白血球＝leukocyte

□ 208

leukemoid reaction 類白血病反応
【luːkíːmɔid riækʃən】

<u>Leukocytosis</u> similar to <u>leukemia</u> but of a different <u>etiology</u>.
白血病と類似するが病因が異なる白血球増加.

| 症 候 | | 定 義 |

☐ 209
thrombocytopenia *¹ 血小板減少
【θràmbousàitəpí:niə】

An abnormal decrease in the number of **platelets**.
血小板の数の異常な減少．

> *1 thrombocytopenia 名 血小板減少
> ⇔ thrombocytosis 名 血小板増加

☐ 210
hemorrhagic diathesis 出血性素因
【hèmərǽdʒik daiǽθəsis】

Abnormally increased tendency toward bleeding.
異常に亢進した出血傾向．

☐ 211
hypercoagulable state *¹ 凝固亢進状態
【háipərkouǽgjuləbl stéit】

Abnormally increased tendency toward **thrombus** formation.
異常に亢進した血栓形成傾向．

> *1 hypercoagulable 形 凝固亢進の ⇔ coagulate 動 凝固する

☐ 212
hyperviscosity 過粘稠度
【háipərviskásəti】

Excessive thickness of blood, usually due to increased amounts of IgM.
血液の粘度の過剰．通常はIgMの増加による．

Chapter 9 Vocabulary

9 血液と造血

Chapter9に収載している医学関連用語の一覧です

英語	日本語
etiology	病因
hemoglobin	ヘモグロビン
leukemia	白血病
leukocytosis	白血球増加

英語	日本語
platelet	血小板
red blood cell	赤血球
thrombus	血栓
white blood cell	白血球

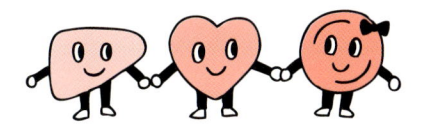

Chapter

10 泌尿器系
Urinary System
【jú(ə)rənèri sístəm】

解剖図

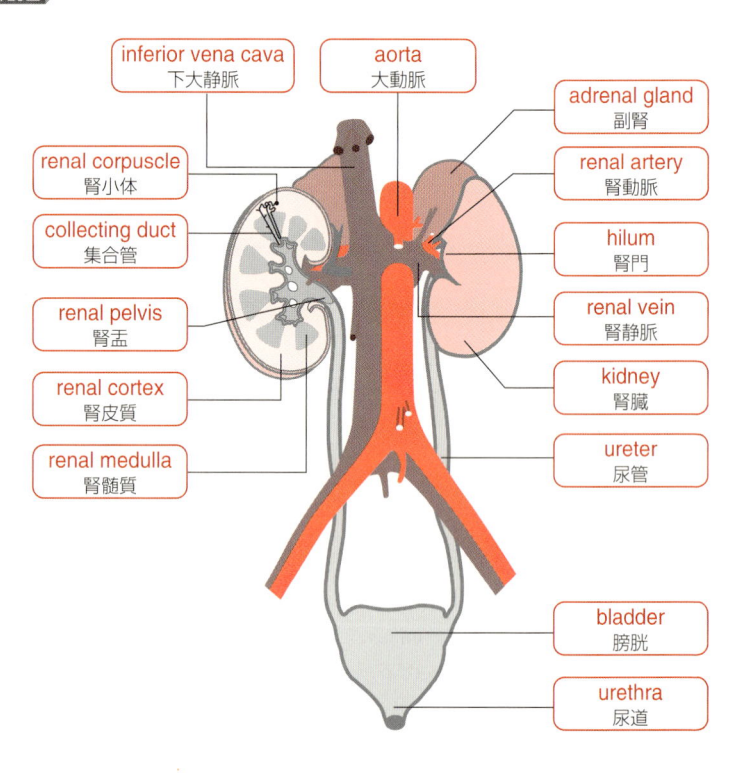

- inferior vena cava 下大静脈
- aorta 大動脈
- adrenal gland 副腎
- renal corpuscle 腎小体
- renal artery 腎動脈
- collecting duct 集合管
- hilum 腎門
- renal pelvis 腎盂
- renal vein 腎静脈
- renal cortex 腎皮質
- kidney 腎臓
- renal medulla 腎髄質
- ureter 尿管
- bladder 膀胱
- urethra 尿道

その症候、英語で言えますか？

10 泌尿器系

症候 | **定義**

213
anuria 　無尿
【ənjú(ə)riə】

Absence of <u>urine</u> formation, clinically defined as output of less than 100 mL per day.

<u>尿</u>が生成されないこと．臨床的には1日100 mL以下の尿量と定義される．

214
oliguria 　乏尿
【àligjú(ə)riə】

Reduced <u>excretion</u> of <u>urine</u>, usually applied to less than 400 mL per day.

<u>尿</u>の<u>排泄</u>の減少．通常は1日400 mL以下のものをいう．

215
polyuria 　多尿
【pàlijú(ə)riə】

Excessive <u>excretion</u> of <u>urine</u>, usually applied to more than 2,500 mL per day.

<u>尿</u>の<u>排泄</u>の過剰．通常は1日2,500 mL以上のものをいう．

216
urinary frequency 　頻尿
【jú(ə)rənèri frí:kwənsi】

Frequent <u>urination</u> at least every two hours during waking hours.

覚醒時における，最低2時間おきの頻繁な<u>排尿</u>．

217
nocturia 　夜間頻尿
【naktjú(ə)riə】

Interruption of sleep one or more times at night to urinate.

排尿のため夜間に1回以上睡眠が中断すること．

症候		定義

218
dysuria
【dìsjú(ə)riə】

排尿痛

Burning or tingling sensation in the <u>urethra</u> or suprapubic*¹ area during or immediately after <u>urination</u>.

<u>排尿</u>の最中または直後の<u>尿道</u>や恥骨上部の灼熱感や刺激感.

* 1 suprapubic 形 恥骨上の ← pubic 形 恥骨の
  ← pubis 名 恥骨

219
urinary retention
【jú(ə)rənèri riténʃən】

尿閉

The inability to pass <u>urine</u> from the <u>bladder</u>.
<u>膀胱</u>から<u>尿</u>を排出できないこと.

220
urinary urgency
【jú(ə)rənèri ə́ːrʤənsi】

尿意切迫

A sudden, strong need to urinate.
突然の強い尿意.

221
urinary incontinence
【jú(ə)rənèri inkántənəns】

尿失禁

The inability to keep <u>urine</u> from leaking from the <u>urethra</u>.
<u>尿</u>が<u>尿道</u>から漏れるのを止められないこと.

222
nocturnal enuresis*¹
【nɑktə́ːrnl ènju(ə)ríːsis】

夜尿症

Involuntary discharge of <u>urine</u> during sleep.
睡眠中の不随意な<u>尿</u>の排出.

* 1 nocturnal enuresis 名 夜尿症
  ⇔ diurnal enuresis 名 昼間遺尿症

10 泌尿器系

症候 / 定義

223
double voiding 二段排尿
[dʌ́bl vɔ́idiŋ]

Having to urinate a second time due to incomplete emptying of the **bladder**.
膀胱が完全に空にならないため，2回目の排尿をしなければならないこと．

224
urinary fistula 尿瘻
[júə(ə)rənèri físʧulə]

An abnormal passage connecting with the **urinary tract**.
尿路とつながっている異常な導管．

225
proteinuria 蛋白尿
[pròutənjúə(ə)riə]

Presence of **urinary protein** in amounts exceeding 150 mg over a 24-hour period.
尿蛋白の量が24時間に150 mgを超えること．

226
glycosuria 糖尿
[glàikousjúə(ə)riə]

Excretion of more than 500 mg of **glucose** in the **urine** per day.
1日あたり500 mgを超えるブドウ糖の尿中への排泄．

227
bilirubinuria ビリルビン尿
[biliru:binjúə(ə)riə]

Excretion of **bilirubin** in the **urine** that indicates an increase of **conjugated bilirubin**[1] levels in blood.
尿中へのビリルビンの排泄．血中の抱合型ビリルビン濃度の上昇を示唆する．

> [1] conjugated bilirubin 名 抱合型ビリルビン
> ⇔ unconjugated bilirubin 名 非抱合型ビリルビン

症候		定義

228

hematuria 血尿
【hìːmətjúəriə】

Presence of blood in the urine that is classified as **gross hematuria** or **microscopic hematuria**.

尿中に血液が存在することで，肉眼的血尿と顕微鏡的血尿に分類される．

229

pyuria 膿尿
【paijúəriə】

Presence of an excessive number of **white blood cells** in the **urine**.

尿中に過剰な数の白血球が存在すること．

230

hemoglobinuria 血色素尿
【hìːməglòubinjúəriə】

Presence of **hemoglobin** in the **urine** that indicates **intravascular**[*1] **hemolysis**[*2].

尿中にヘモグロビンが存在することで，血管内溶血を示唆する．

*1 intravascular 形 血管内の ← vascular 形 血管の
*2 hemolysis 名 溶血

231

myoglobinuria ミオグロビン尿
【maiougloubinjúəriə】

Presence of **myoglobin** in the **urine**, usually associated with muscle **necrosis**.

尿中にミオグロビンが存在することで，通常は筋肉の壊死に関連する．

232

chyluria 乳び尿
【kailjúəriə】

Presence of **chyle** in the **urine** due to **obstruction** of **lymphatic vessels** by **parasites** or **tumor cells**.

尿中に乳糜が存在することで，寄生虫または腫瘍細胞によるリンパ管の閉塞に起因する．

Chapter 10 Vocabulary

Chapter10に収載している医学関連用語の一覧です

英語	日本語
bilirubin	ビリルビン
bladder	膀胱
chyle	乳糜
conjugated bilirubin	抱合型ビリルビン
excretion	排泄
glucose	ブドウ糖
gross hematuria	肉眼的血尿
hemoglobin	ヘモグロビン
intravascular hemolysis	血管内溶血
lymphatic vessel	リンパ管
microscopic hematuria	顕微鏡的血尿
myoglobin	ミオグロビン
necrosis	壊死
obstruction	閉塞
parasite	寄生虫
tumor cell	腫瘍細胞
urethra	尿道
urinary protein	尿蛋白
urinary tract	尿路
urination	排尿
urine	尿
white blood cell	白血球

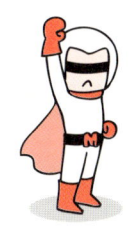

Chapter 11

生殖器系
Reproductive System
[rìːprədʌ́ktiv sístəm]

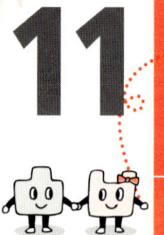

解剖図

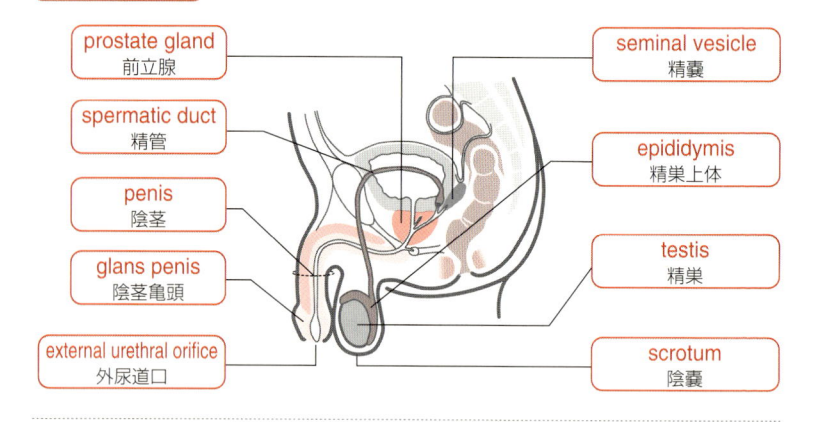

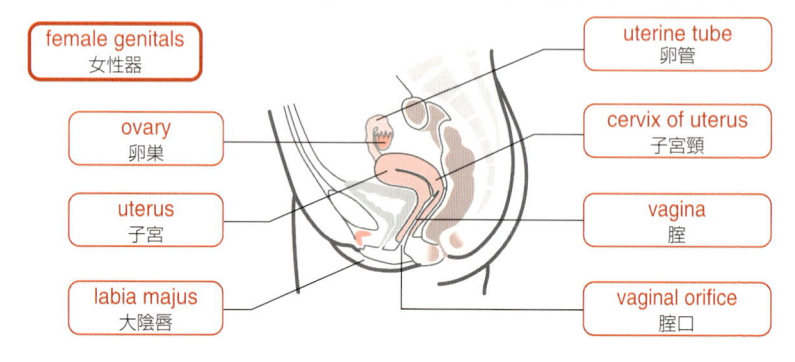

- male genitals / 男性器
  - prostate gland / 前立腺
  - spermatic duct / 精管
  - penis / 陰茎
  - glans penis / 陰茎亀頭
  - external urethral orifice / 外尿道口
  - seminal vesicle / 精囊
  - epididymis / 精巣上体
  - testis / 精巣
  - scrotum / 陰囊

- female genitals / 女性器
  - ovary / 卵巣
  - uterus / 子宮
  - labia majus / 大陰唇
  - uterine tube / 卵管
  - cervix of uterus / 子宮頸
  - vagina / 腟
  - vaginal orifice / 腟口

その症候、英語で言えますか？

11 生殖器系

| 症候 | 定義 |

233
hematospermia 血精液症
[hiːmətouspéːmiə]

Presence of blood in <u>seminal fluid</u> that is usually benign and idiopathic[*1].

<u>精液</u>中に血液が存在することで，通常は良性で特発性である．

* 1 idiopathic 形 特発性の

234
uterine[*1] **prolapse** 子宮脱
[júːtərin próulæps]

Downward displacement of the <u>uterus</u> due to <u>laxity</u> of the muscular and fascial[*2] structures of the <u>pelvic</u>[*3] <u>floor</u>.

骨盤底の筋肉および筋膜構造の<u>弛緩</u>による<u>子宮</u>の下方への移動．

* 1 uterine 形 子宮の ← uterus 名 子宮
* 2 fascial 形 筋膜の ← fascia 名 筋膜
* 3 pelvic 形 骨盤の ← pelvis 名 骨盤

235
cystocele 膀胱瘤
[sístəsìːl]

A <u>hernia</u> of the <u>bladder</u> protruding into the <u>vagina</u>.

<u>膣</u>に脱出している<u>膀胱</u>の<u>ヘルニア</u>．

236
leukorrhea 白帯下
[lùːkəríːə]

Discharge from the <u>vagina</u> of a white or yellowish viscid[*1] fluid containing <u>mucus</u> and <u>pus cells</u>.

<u>粘液</u>および<u>膿細胞</u>を含む白色または黄色で粘着性の液体を<u>膣</u>から排出すること．

* 1 viscid 形 粘着性の

症 候		定 義

237

dysmenorrhea 月経困難
【dìsmenərí:ə】

Intermittent[*1], cramping pain felt in the lower abdomen during menstruation, sometimes accompanied by nausea or headache.

月経期間中に下腹部に感じる断続的な痙攣痛で，悪心または頭痛を伴うこともある．

＊1 intermittent 形 断続的な

238

mittelschmerz 中間痛
【mítlʃmèərts】

Pain felt in the ovary area at the time of ovulation around the midpoint of the menstrual[*1] cycle.

月経周期のほぼ中間にあたる排卵の時期に卵巣部分に感じる痛み．

＊1 menstrual 形 月経の ← menstruation 名 月経

239

amenorrhea 無月経
【eimènərí:ə】

Absence of menarche by age 18, or abnormal cessation of menstruation.

18歳までに初経がないこと．または月経の異常な停止．

240

polymenorrhea 頻発月経
【pàlimenərí:ə】

Abnormally frequent menstruation at intervals of less than 21 days.

異常に頻度の多い月経で，間隔が21日未満のものをいう．

11 生殖器系

症候 | **定義**

☐ 241
oligomenorrhea 希発月経
【àligoumenərí:ə】

Abnormally infrequent **menstruation** at intervals of greater than 35 days.

異常に頻度の少ない月経で，間隔が35日を超えるものをいう．

☐ 242
hypermenorrhea *1 月経過多
【hàipərmenərí:ə】

Abnormally profuse or prolonged **uterine bleeding** during **menstruation**.

月経中の過量または過長な子宮出血．

＊1　hypermenorrhea 名月経過多 ⇔ hypomenorrhea 名月経過少

☐ 243
metrorrhagia 不正子宮出血
【metrəræʤiə】

Uterine bleeding at irregular intervals that is not associated with **menstruation**.

月経と関係のない不規則な間隔の子宮出血．

☐ 244
infertility 不妊
【infərtíləti】

The inability to achieve **conception** after one year of regular **intercourse** without **contraception**.

避妊をせずに1年間の定期的な性交を経ても受胎が起こらないこと．

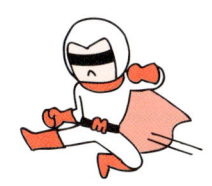

| 症 候 | 定 義 |

☐ 245

hyperemesis gravidarum *1
【háipərémǝsis grævǝdé(ǝ)rǝm】

妊娠悪阻

Excessive **nausea** and **vomiting** commonly seen in the first 12 weeks of **pregnancy**.

一般に妊娠12週までにみられる過度の悪心および嘔吐.

* 1 hyperemesis gravidarum 名 妊娠悪阻 = morning sickness 名 つわり

☐ 246

abortion
【ǝbɔ́:rʃǝn】

流産

Expulsion of a nonviable *1 **embryo** or **fetus** from the **uterus**.

子宮から成育不可能な胎芽または胎児を娩出すること.

* 1 nonviable 形 成育不可能な ⇔ viable 形 成育可能な

☐ 247

premature birth
【pri:mǝtʃúǝr bə́:rθ】

早産

Childbirth occurring earlier than 37 completed weeks of **gestation**. *1

妊娠満37週未満の出産.

* 1 gestation 名 妊娠 = pregnancy

☐ 248

precocious puberty
【prikóuʃǝs pjú:bǝrti】

思春期早発症

The appearance of **signs** of pubertal *1 development before age 7 or 8 in girls and age 9 in boys.

思春期発達の徴候が女児では7〜8歳未満, 男児では9歳未満に出現すること.

* 1 pubertal 形 思春期の ⇐ puberty 名 思春期

11 生殖器系

症候 | **定義**

☐ 249
delayed puberty 思春期遅発症
【diléid pjú:bərti】

Lack of any <u>signs</u> of <u>puberty</u> by age 14 in either sex.
男女いずれにおいても14歳までに**思春期**の<u>徴候</u>がみられないこと．

☐ 250
premature ejaculation 早漏
【prì:mətʃúər idʒæ̀kjuléiʃən】

<u>Ejaculation</u> during the early stages of <u>sexual excitement</u>.
<u>性的興奮</u>の初期段階での<u>射精</u>．

☐ 251
retrograde ejaculation 逆行性射精
【rétrəgrèid idʒæ̀kjuléiʃən】

Entry of <u>seminal fluid</u> into the <u>bladder</u> during <u>ejaculation</u>.
<u>射精</u>時に<u>精液</u>が<u>膀胱</u>に流入すること．

☐ 252
erectile dysfunction 勃起不全
【iréktail disfʌ́ŋkʃən】

The inability to obtain penile[*1] rigidity sufficient for <u>intercourse</u>.
<u>性交</u>に十分な陰茎の硬度が得られないこと．

*1 penile 形 陰茎の ← penis 名 陰茎

Chapter 11 Vocabulary

Chapter11に収載している医学関連用語の一覧です

英語	日本語
bladder	膀胱
childbirth	出産
conception	受胎
contraception	避妊
cramping pain	痙攣痛
ejaculation	射精
embryo	胎芽
fetus	胎児
gestation	妊娠
headache	頭痛
hernia	ヘルニア
intercourse	性交
laxity	弛緩
lower abdomen	下腹部
menarche	初経
menstrual cycle	月経周期

英語	日本語
menstruation	月経
mucus	粘液
nausea	悪心
ovary	卵巣
ovulation	排卵
pelvic floor	骨盤底
pregnancy	妊娠
puberty	思春期
pus cell	膿細胞
seminal fluid	精液
sexual excitement	性的興奮
sign	徴候
uterine bleeding	子宮出血
uterus	子宮
vagina	膣
vomiting	嘔吐

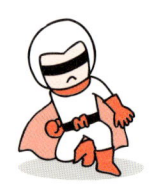

Chapter 12

精神機能
Mental Function
【méntl fʌ́ŋkʃən】

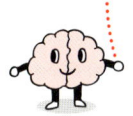

症候 / 定義

253
dementia 認知症
【diménʃiə】

Loss of cognitive*¹ and intellectual functions without impairment of **perception** or **consciousness**.
認知および知的機能の喪失で，知覚や意識の障害は伴わない．

*1 cognitive 形 認知の ← cognition 名 認知

254
pseudodementia 仮性認知症
【súːdou-diménʃiə】

Dementia due to a **mood disorder** rather than **brain dysfunction**.
脳機能障害ではなく気分障害に起因する認知症．

255
amnesia 健忘
【æmníːziə】

Partial or total inability to recall past experiences.
過去の経験を思い出すことが部分的または完全にできないこと．

256
Korsakoff syndrome コルサコフ症候群
【kɔ́ːrsəkɔːf síndroum】

Mental impairment characterized by **disorientation**, **amnesia**, and **confabulation**.
見当識障害，健忘，作話を特徴とする精神障害．

| 症 候 | | 定 義 |

□ 257
mental retardation 精神遅滞 Subnormal intellectual development accompanied by impairment in **adaptive behavior**.
【méntl riːtɑːrdéiʃən】
適応行動の障害を伴う正常以下の知的発達.

□ 258
disorientation 見当識障害 Confusion in recognition of time, place, and person.
【disɔ̀ːriəntéiʃən】
時間，場所，人の認識における混乱.

□ 259
illusion 錯覚 A misperception of **external stimuli** *1.
【ilúːʒən】
外部刺激を誤って知覚すること.

> ＊1 stimuli 名 刺激（複数形；単数形は stimulus）

□ 260
hallucination 幻覚 A subjective perception of **stimuli** that do not exist.
【həlùːsənéiʃən】
存在しない刺激を主観的に知覚すること.

□ 261
delusion 妄想 A false belief that is firmly maintained despite evidence to the contrary.
【dilúːʒən】
反対の証拠があるにもかかわらず強固に維持される誤った信念.

□ 262
obsession 強迫 An irrational thought or **impulse** that recurs and persists despite attempts to suppress it.
【əbséʃən】
抑えようと試みても繰り返し現れて持続する不合理な考えや衝動.

12 精神機能

症候		定義

☐ 263
anxiety
【æŋzáiəti】

不安

Experience of fear or apprehension in response to anticipated internal or external danger.

予期される内的または外的な危険に対して恐れや懸念を経験すること．

☐ 264
panic attack
【pǽnik ətǽk】

パニック発作

Sudden onset of intense **anxiety** accompanied by **palpitations**, **shortness of breath**, and **sweating**.

突然に生じる激しい<u>不安</u>で，<u>動悸</u>，<u>息切れ</u>，<u>発汗</u>を伴う．

☐ 265
phobia
【fóubiə】

恐怖症

An irrational and intense fear of a specific object or situation.

ある特定の物体や状況に対する不合理な激しい恐れ．

☐ 266
depressive state
【diprésiv stéit】

うつ状態

A mental state characterized by feelings of sadness, loneliness, despair, low self-esteem, and self-reproach.

悲しみ，孤独，絶望，自尊心の低下，自責感を特徴とする精神状態．

☐ 267
manic state
【mǽnik stéit】

躁状態

A distinct period of persistently elevated and expansive mood.

高揚した誇大的な気分が一定期間持続している状態．

症候		定義

☐ 268

ambivalence 両価性 The coexistence of opposing attitudes or emotions toward a person or a thing.
【æmbívələns】

ある人や物に対して相反する態度や情動が共存すること．

☐ 269

depersonalization 離人症 An alteration in the perception of the self where the normal sense of personal reality is lost.
【di:pə̀:rsənəlaizéiʃən】

自己の認識が変容し，正常な個人的現実感が失われた状態．

☐ 270

conversion 転換 A psychological [*1] **defense mechanism** by which unconscious **conflict** or repressed thought is transformed into bodily **symptoms**.
【kənvə́:rʒən】

無意識の**葛藤**や抑圧された考えが身体的な**症状**に変換される心理的**防衛機制**．

[*1] psychological 形 心理的な ← psychology 名 心理，心理学

☐ 271

delusion of control させられ体験 A false belief that some external force controls one's feelings, thoughts, or actions.
【dilú:ʒən əv kəntróul】

ある外部の力が自分の感情，思考，行動をコントロールしているという誤った信念．

症候		定義

272
catatonia
【kætətóuniə】

緊張病

Psychomotor*¹ disturbance characterized by physical **rigidity** and **stupor**.

身体**硬直**と**昏迷**を特徴とする精神運動障害.

＊1 psychomotor 形 精神運動の

273
attention deficit hyperactivity disorder (ADHD)
【əténʃən défəsit hàipəræktívəti disɔ́:rdər】

注意欠陥多動性障害

A behavioral developmental disorder*¹,² characterized by **inattentiveness**, **impulsiveness**, and **hyperactivity**.

注意散漫，**衝動性**，**多動性**を特徴とする行動・発達障害.

＊1 behavioral disorder 名 行動障害
＊2 developmental disorder 名 発達障害

274
distractibility
【distræktəbíləti】

転導性

An **attention disorder** in which the mind is easily diverted by irrelevant **stimuli**.

無関係の**刺激**により容易に気が散ってしまう**注意障害**.

275
abulia
【eibú:liə】

無為

Loss or impairment of the ability to perform voluntary actions or to make decisions.

自発的行動や決定を行う能力の喪失または障害.

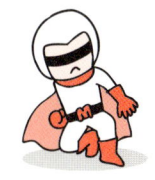

| 症候 | | 定義 |

□ 276
autism　自閉
【ɔ́ːtizm】

Abnormal <u>self-absorption</u> characterized by lack of response to people and limited ability to communicate.

人に対する反応の欠如と限られたコミュニケーション能力を特徴とする異常な**自己専心**.

□ 277
insomnia　不眠
【insámniə】

Chronic inability to fall asleep or remain asleep for an adequate length of time.

慢性的に眠りにつけない状態，または十分な時間睡眠を継続できない状態.

□ 278
hypersomnia　過眠
【hàipərsámniə】

Excessive daytime sleepiness or sleep of excessive duration.

過剰な日中の眠気または極端に長い睡眠.

□ 279
hypochondriasis　心気症
【hàipoukəndráiəsis】

A morbid[*1] concern about one's own health or excessive <u>anxiety</u> about having a serious illness.

自分の健康に関する病的な懸念または重病にかかっているという過剰な**不安**.

＊1 morbid 形 病的な

□ 280
aphasia　失語
【əféiʒiə】

A partial or total loss of the ability to comprehend or produce language.

言語を理解または産出する能力が一部またはすべて失われること．

症候		定義

281

paraphasia 錯語
【pærəféiʒiə】

Production of unintended syllables, words, or phrases during speech.

発話中に意図しない音節，単語，フレーズを話してしまうこと．

282

Broca's aphasia[*1] ブローカ失語
【bróukəz əféiʒiə】

Impairment in language production characterized by reduced speech output, word-finding difficulties, and impaired repetition.

発話量の減少，換語困難，復唱の障害を特徴とする言語産出の障害．

[*1] Broca's aphasia 名 ブローカ失語 = motor aphasia 名 運動性失語

283

Wernicke's aphasia[*1] ウェルニッケ失語
【və́:rnikiz əféiʒiə】

Impairment in the comprehension of spoken and written words accompanied by **paraphasia**.

話し言葉や書き言葉の理解における障害で，<u>錯語</u>を伴う．

[*1] Wernicke's aphasia 名 ウェルニッケ失語 = sensory aphasia 名 感覚性失語

284

apraxia 失行
【əpræksiə】

A partial or total loss of the ability to perform purposeful acts or learned movements without motor or sensory impairment.

意図的な行為や学習した動きを行う能力が一部またはすべて失われること．運動や感覚の障害はない．

症候		定義

285
agnosia
【ægnóuʒə】

失認

Impairment of the ability to recognize or comprehend various **sensory stimuli** such as objects, people, sounds, shapes, and smells.

物体，人，音，形，においなどのさまざまな**感覚刺激**を認識したり理解したりする能力の障害．

286
Gerstmann syndrome
【gə́:rstmɑ:n síndroum】

ゲルストマン症候群

A **neurological**[*1] **disorder** characterized by **finger agnosia**, **right-left agnosia**, **agraphia**, and **acalculia**.

手指失認，**左右失認**，**失書**，**失算**を特徴とする**神経障害**．

> *1 neurological 形 神経の，神経学の ← neurology 名 神経学

287
vegetative state
【védʒətèitiv stéit】

植物状態

Absence of **cognitive function** with preserved ability to maintain **blood pressure**, **respiration**, and **cardiac function**.

認知機能は喪失しているが，**血圧**，**呼吸**，**心臓機能**を維持する能力は保たれている状態．

288
akinetic[*1] **mutism**
【eikinétic mjú:tizm】

無動無言症

A persistent state of **altered consciousness** characterized by the inability to speak and loss of voluntary movement.

話す能力の欠如および随意行動の喪失を特徴とする持続性の**意識変容**状態．

> *1 akinetic 形 無動の ← akinesia 名 無動

12 精神機能

症 候		定 義

□ 289
locked-in syndrome　閉じ込め症候群
【lákt-in síndroum】

A **neurological disorder** with preserved **consciousness** characterized by **tetraplegia***1, **dysphagia**, and facial **diplegia**.

意識が保たれている**神経障害**で，**四肢麻痺**，**嚥下障害**，顔面**両側麻痺**を特徴とする．

*1 tetraplegia 名 四肢麻痺＝ quadriplegia

□ 290
somnolence　傾眠
【sámnələns】

The inability to maintain an adequate level of **wakefulness**.

適切な**覚醒**の程度を維持できないこと．

□ 291
stupor　昏迷
【st(j)úːpər】

A marked diminution in reactivity to **environmental stimuli** that can be aroused only by vigorous stimulation.

環境刺激に対する反応の著しい減退で，強度の刺激によってのみ覚醒させることができる．

□ 292
coma　昏睡
【kóumə】

A state of deep **unconsciousness** in which an individual is incapable of sensing or responding to **external stimuli** and **internal needs**.

外部刺激および**内的欲求**を感じたりそれらに反応したりすることができない深い**無意識**の状態．

症候		定義

293

delirium   せん妄   Acute disorder of <u>attention</u> and <u>cognitive function</u> combined with <u>hallucinations</u> and <u>delusions</u>.
【dilíriəm】

注意および認知機能の急性障害で，幻覚や妄想を伴う．

294

confusion   錯乱   <u>Disturbance of consciousness</u> characterized by lack of orderly thought.
【kənfjúːʒən】

筋道の通った思考の欠如を特徴とする意識障害．

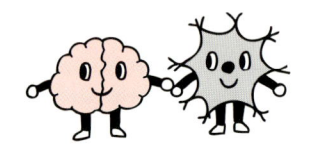

Chapter 12 Vocabulary

Chapter12に収載している医学関連用語の一覧です

英語	日本語
acalculia	失算
adaptive behavior	適応行動
agraphia	失書
altered consciousness	意識変容
amnesia	健忘
anxiety	不安
attention	注意
attention disorder	注意障害
blood pressure	血圧
brain dysfunction	脳機能障害
cardiac function	心臓機能
cognitive function	認知機能
confabulation	作話
conflict	葛藤
consciousness	意識
defense mechanism	防衛機制
delusion	妄想
dementia	認知症
diplegia	両側麻痺
disorientation	見当識障害
disturbance of consciousness	意識障害
dysphagia	嚥下障害
environmental stimuli	環境刺激
external stimuli	外部刺激
finger agnosia	手指失認

英語	日本語
hallucination	幻覚
hyperactivity	多動性
impulse	衝動
impulsiveness	衝動性
inattentiveness	注意散漫
internal need	内的欲求
mental impairment	精神障害
mood disorder	気分障害
neurological disorder	神経障害
palpitation	動悸
paraphasia	錯語
perception	知覚
respiration	呼吸
right-left agnosia	左右失認
rigidity	硬直
self-absorption	自己専心
sensory stimuli	感覚刺激
shortness of breath	息切れ
stimuli (stimulus)	刺激
stupor	昏迷
sweating	発汗
symptom	症状
tetraplegia	四肢麻痺
unconsciousness	無意識
wakefulness	覚醒

Chapter 13

神経系
Nervous System
【né:rvəs sístəm】

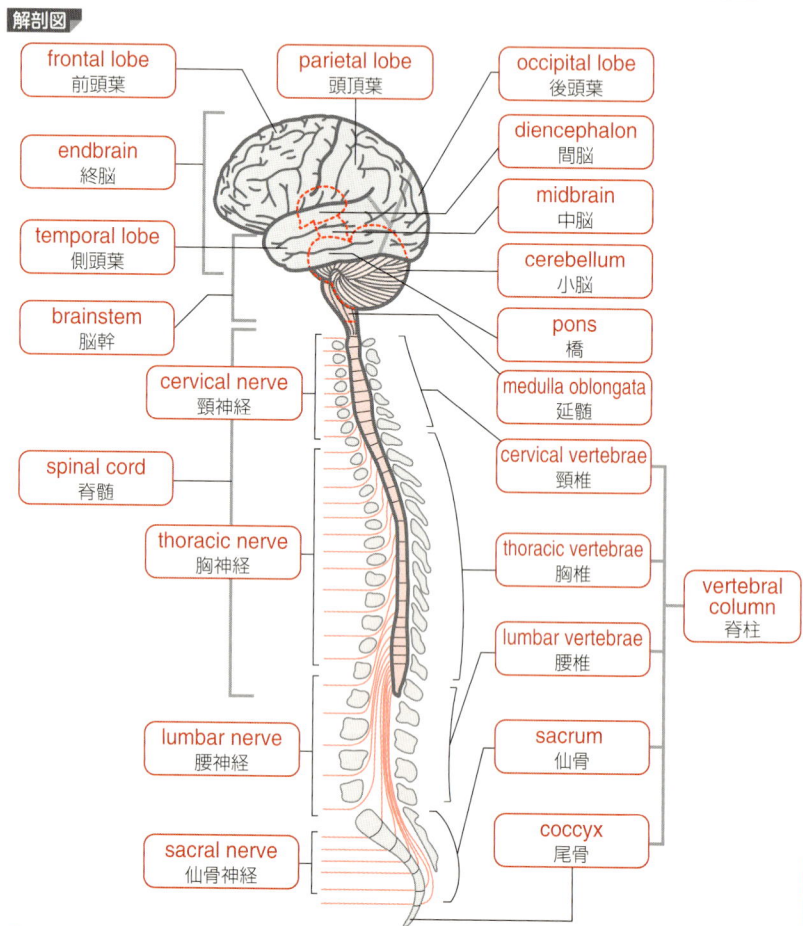

解剖図

- frontal lobe 前頭葉
- parietal lobe 頭頂葉
- occipital lobe 後頭葉
- endbrain 終脳
- diencephalon 間脳
- midbrain 中脳
- temporal lobe 側頭葉
- cerebellum 小脳
- brainstem 脳幹
- pons 橋
- cervical nerve 頸神経
- medulla oblongata 延髄
- spinal cord 脊髄
- cervical vertebrae 頸椎
- thoracic nerve 胸神経
- thoracic vertebrae 胸椎
- lumbar vertebrae 腰椎
- vertebral column 脊柱
- lumbar nerve 腰神経
- sacrum 仙骨
- sacral nerve 仙骨神経
- coccyx 尾骨

その症候、英語で言えますか？

症 候		定 義

☐ 295
Horner syndrome
【hɔ́:rnər síndroum】

ホルネル症候群

Ipsilateral[*1] **miosis**, **blepharoptosis**, and facial **anhidrosis** due to a **lesion** of the **cervical**[*2] **sympathetic chain**.

頸部交感神経鎖の病変による同側の縮瞳，眼瞼下垂，および顔面無汗症．

*1 ipsilateral 形 同側の
*2 cervical 形 頸部の ← cervix 名 頸部

☐ 296
Adie syndrome
【éidi síndroum】

アディー症候群

A **neurological disorder** characterized by **mydriasis** and loss of deep **tendon reflexes**.

散瞳と深部腱反射の消失を特徴とする神経障害．

☐ 297
Argyll Robertson pupil
【ɑ:rgáil rábərtsn pjú:pil】

アーガイル・ロバートソン瞳孔

A form of **pupillary rigidity** characterized by **miosis** and loss of **light reflex**, often seen in **tabetic neurosyphilis**.

縮瞳および対光反射の消失を特徴とする瞳孔強直の一種で，しばしば脊髄癆性神経梅毒にみられる．

☐ 298
Bell's palsy
【bélz pɔ́:lzi】

ベル麻痺

Usually unilateral[*1] **paralysis** of the **facial muscles** caused by **dysfunction** of the **seventh cranial nerve**[*2].

第七脳神経の機能障害による通常は片側の顔面筋の麻痺．

*1 unilateral 形 片側の
*2 seventh cranial nerve 名 第七脳神経＝ facial nerve 名 顔面神経

症候		定義

299
dysarthria 構音障害
[disá:rθriə]

Difficulty in articulating *1 words due to **paralysis**, **incoordination**, or **spasticity** of **speech muscles**.

発話筋の麻痺，協調運動障害，または痙縮による語の発音困難．

*1 articulate 動 発音する

300
Kernig sign ケルニヒ徴候
[kə́:rnig sáin]

A **clinical sign** of **meningitis** that consists of pain and resistance on attempting to extend the leg with the **thigh** flexed at the **hip joint**.

髄膜炎の臨床徴候のひとつで，大腿を股関節で屈曲した状態で下肢を伸ばそうとすると痛みや抵抗を伴う．

301
Brudzinski sign ブルジンスキー徴候
[bruʤínski sáin]

Involuntary flexion of the **knee joints** and **hip joints** following flexion of the neck while supine *1.

仰臥位での首の屈曲に伴う膝関節と股関節の不随意な屈曲．

*1 supine 形 仰臥の

302
nuchal *1 rigidity 項部硬直
[njú:kəl riʤídəti]

Impaired neck flexion due to **spasm** of the **extensor muscles** of the neck.

首の伸筋の痙攣による首屈曲の障害．

*1 nuchal 形 項部の ← nucha 名 項部

13 神経系

症候 / 定義

303

megacephaly 大頭症
【mégəséfəli】

Congenital*¹ or acquired*² condition of having an abnormally large <u>cranial capacity</u>.

異常に大きな<u>頭蓋容量</u>を呈する先天性または後天性の症状.

* 1 congenital 形 先天性の
* 2 acquired 形 後天性の

304

microcephaly 小頭症
【maikrouséfəli】

Abnormally small <u>cranium</u>, usually associated with <u>mental retardation</u>.

異常に小さい<u>頭蓋</u>. 通常, <u>精神遅滞</u>を伴う.

305

craniosynostosis 頭蓋縫合早期癒合症
【krèiniousinəstóusis】

Premature closure of <u>cranial sutures</u> resulting in <u>malformation</u> of the <u>cranium</u>.

<u>頭蓋</u>の<u>奇形</u>を生じる<u>頭蓋縫合</u>の早期の癒合.

306

spasticity 痙縮
【spæstísəti】

Increase in <u>muscle tone</u> at rest, characterized by resistance to passive stretch.

安静時の<u>筋緊張</u>の亢進. 受動的な伸展に対する抵抗を特徴とする.

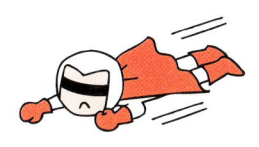

症候		定義

☐ **307**

Babinski sign
【bəbínski sáin】

バビンスキー徴候

Dorsiflexion of the great toe and abduction of the other toes to plantar*¹ stimulation, indicative of pyramidal tract involvement.

足底刺激による拇趾の背屈および他の趾の外転．錐体路障害を示唆する．

＊1 plantar 形 足底の

☐ **308**

Chaddock reflex
【tʃǽdək ríːfleks】

チャドック反射

Dorsiflexion of the great toe to stimulation of the skin over the lateral*¹ malleolus.

外側くるぶしの皮膚刺激による拇趾の背屈．

＊1 lateral 形 外側の，側方の

☐ **309**

dystonia
【distóuniə】

ジストニア

Abnormal tonicity of muscle characterized by prolonged, repetitive contractions.

持続時間の長い反復性の収縮を特徴とする筋肉の異常な緊張．

☐ **310**

tremor
【trémər】

振戦

Rhythmic involuntary movements caused by alternate contraction of opposing muscle groups.

対立筋群の交互の収縮により生じる律動性の不随意運動．

☐ **311**

chorea
【kəríːə】

舞踏運動

Spasmodic involuntary movements of the limbs or facial muscles.

四肢や顔面筋の痙攣性の不随意運動．

13 神経系

症候 | *定義*

□ 312

myoclonus
【maiáklənəs】

ミオクローヌス　Brief involuntary <u>contractions</u> of a single muscle or muscle group that are of variable regularity, synchrony, and symmetry.

単一筋または筋群の短い不随意<u>収縮</u>．規則性，同期性，対称性は変化に富む．

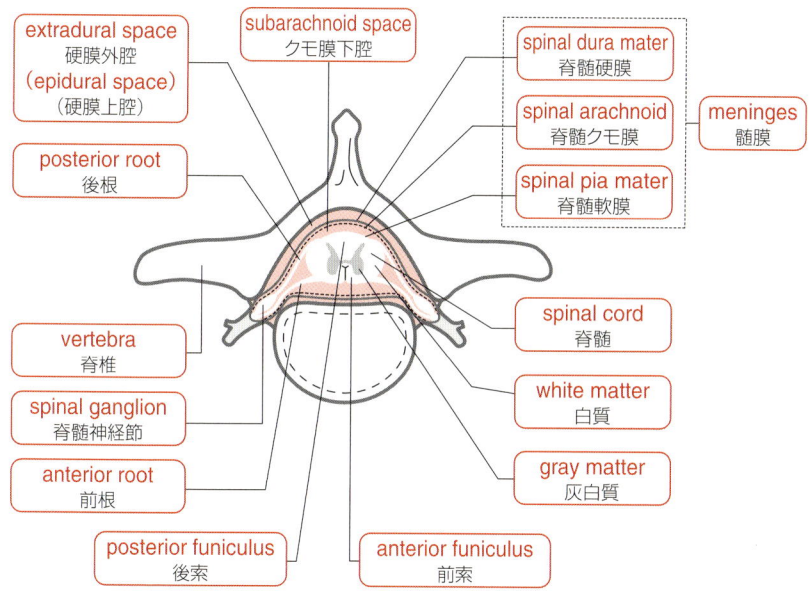

- extradural space 硬膜外腔 (epidural space)（硬膜上腔）
- subarachnoid space クモ膜下腔
- spinal dura mater 脊髄硬膜
- spinal arachnoid 脊髄クモ膜
- spinal pia mater 脊髄軟膜
- meninges 髄膜
- posterior root 後根
- vertebra 脊椎
- spinal ganglion 脊髄神経節
- anterior root 前根
- spinal cord 脊髄
- white matter 白質
- gray matter 灰白質
- posterior funiculus 後索
- anterior funiculus 前索

解剖図 脊髄の構造

症候		定義

□ 313
ataxia
【ətǽksiə】

運動失調

The inability to coordinate muscle activity during <u>voluntary movement</u>, usually due to disorders of the <u>cerebellum</u> or the <u>posterior funiculus</u> of the <u>spinal cord</u>.
<u>随意運動</u>中に筋活動を協調させられないこと．通常は<u>小脳</u>または<u>脊髄</u>の<u>後索</u>の疾患による．

□ 314
Romberg sign
【rάmbə:rg sáin】

ロンベルク徴候

Unsteadiness of the body when standing erect with feet together and eyes closed.
両足をそろえ眼を閉じて直立した際の身体の不安定．

□ 315
hypesthesia
【hìpəsθí:ziə】

感覚鈍麻

Decreased <u>sensitivity</u> to touch and pain.
接触や痛みに対する<u>感受性</u>の低下．

□ 316
paresthesia
【pæ̀rəsθí:ziə】

感覚異常

Abnormal sensations, such as <u>numbness</u> or <u>tingling</u>, in the <u>extremities</u> in the absence of <u>stimuli</u>.
<u>刺激</u>が存在しない状態での<u>四肢</u>における<u>しびれ</u>や<u>刺痛</u>等の異常な感覚．

□ 317
retropulsion
【rètrəpʌ́lʒən】

後方突進

An involuntary backward walking or running, associated especially with <u>Parkinson's disease</u>.
不随意な後方への歩行または走行．主に<u>パーキンソン病</u>に関連する．

13 神経系

症候 / 定義

□ 318
orthostatic hypotension
【ɔ̀ːrθəstǽtik hàipouténʃən】
起立性低血圧

A drop in **blood pressure** upon assuming the standing position, accompanied by **dizziness** or **syncope**.

起立姿勢をとった時の血圧の低下．めまい感や失神を伴う．

□ 319
transverse myelopathy
【trænzvə́ːrs màiəlápəθi】
横断性脊髄症

Lesions of the **spinal cord** that extend across the width of the thick cord of **nervous tissue**.

太い神経組織の束を横断するように広がる脊髄の病変．

□ 320
Brown-Sequard syndrome
【bráun-sekáːr síndroum】
ブラウン・セカール症候群

Unilateral **lesions** of the **spinal cord**, resulting in ipsilateral **proprioception** loss and **muscle weakness** as well as contralateral*1 loss of **pain and temperature sensation**.

脊髄の片側の病変で，同側の固有受容感覚喪失および筋力低下，対側の温痛覚喪失を引き起こす．

＊1 contralateral 形 対側の

□ 321
peripheral neuropathy
【pərífərəl njurápəθi】
末梢神経障害

Damage to the **motor nerves** and **sensory nerves**, causing **muscle atrophy**, **muscle weakness**, **hypesthesia**, and **paresthesia**.

運動神経および感覚神経の損傷．筋萎縮，筋力低下，感覚鈍麻，感覚異常を生じる．

症候		定義

□ 322

lordosis 前彎 Abnormal forward <u>curvature</u> of the lumbar[*1] and
【lɔːrdóusis】 cervical regions of the <u>vertebral column</u>.

<u>脊柱</u>の腰部および頸部における異常な前方<u>彎曲</u>.

*1 lumbar 形 腰部の

□ 323

kyphosis 後彎 Abnormal backward <u>curvature</u> of the thoracic[*1]
【kaifóusis】 region of the <u>vertebral column</u>.

<u>脊柱</u>の胸部における異常な後方<u>彎曲</u>.

*1 thoracic 形 胸部の

□ 324

scoliosis 側彎 Abnormal lateral <u>curvature</u> of the <u>vertebral column</u>.
【skòulióusis】
<u>脊柱</u>の異常な側方<u>彎曲</u>.

□ 325

ankylosis 関節強直 Stiffening or fusion of a <u>joint</u> as a result of injury or
【æŋkəlóusis】 disease.

外傷または疾患に起因する<u>関節</u>の硬直または癒合.

Chapter 13 Vocabulary

Chapter13に収載している医学関連用語の一覧です

英語	日本語	英語	日本語
abduction	外転	blood pressure	血圧
anhidrosis	無汗症	cerebellum	小脳
blepharoptosis	眼瞼下垂	cervical sympathetic chain	頸部交感神経鎖

13 神経系

英語	日本語
clinical sign	臨床徴候
contraction	収縮
cranial capacity	頭蓋容量
cranial suture	頭蓋縫合
cranium	頭蓋
curvature	彎曲
dizziness	めまい感
dorsiflexion	背屈
dysfunction	機能障害
extensor muscle	伸筋
extremities	四肢
facial muscle	顔面筋
great toe	拇趾
hip joint	股関節
hypesthesia	感覚鈍麻
incoordination	協調運動障害
involuntary movement	不随意運動
joint	関節
knee joint	膝関節
lesion	病変
light reflex	対光反射
limbs	四肢
malformation	奇形
malleolus	くるぶし
meningitis	髄膜炎
mental retardation	精神遅滞
miosis	縮瞳
motor nerve	運動神経
muscle atrophy	筋萎縮
muscle tone	筋緊張
muscle weakness	筋力低下
mydriasis	散瞳
nervous tissue	神経組織
neurological disorder	神経障害
numbness	しびれ
opposing muscle group	対立筋群
pain and temperature sensation	温痛覚
paralysis	麻痺
paresthesia	感覚異常
Parkinson's disease	パーキンソン病
plantar stimulation	足底刺激
posterior funiculus	後索
proprioception	固有受容感覚
pupillary rigidity	瞳孔強直
pyramidal tract	錐体路
sensitivity	感受性
sensory nerve	感覚神経
seventh cranial nerve	第七脳神経
spasm	痙攣
spasticity	痙縮
speech muscle	発話筋
spinal cord	脊髄
stimuli	刺激
syncope	失神
tabetic neurosyphilis	脊髄癆性神経梅毒
tendon reflex	腱反射
thigh	大腿
tingling	刺痛
tonicity	緊張
vertebral column	脊柱
voluntary movement	随意運動

Chapter 14

内分泌系と代謝
Endocrine System and Metabolism
[éndəkrin sístəm] and [mətǽbəlìzm]

症候		定義

□ 326

gigantism
[dʒaigǽntizm]

巨人症

Excessive growth of the body usually caused by <u>oversecretion</u> of the <u>growth hormone</u> before the <u>epiphyseal lines</u> close.

身体の過剰な成長で,通常は**骨端線**が閉鎖する以前の**成長ホルモン**の**過剰分泌**により生じる.

□ 327

acromegaly
[æ̀kroumégəli]

末端肥大症

Progressive [*1] <u>enlargement</u> of peripheral parts of the body resulting from abnormal activity of the <u>pituitary gland</u>.

下垂体の異常な活動に起因する身体の末梢部の進行性**肥大**.

*1 progressive 形 進行性の

□ 328

virilism
[vírəlìzm]

男性化

The appearance of male <u>secondary sex characteristics</u> in a female caused by excessive production of <u>androgens</u>.

アンドロゲンの過剰産生により女性に男性の**二次性徴**が現れること.

14 内分泌系と代謝

症 候 **定 義**

□ 329
gynecomastia 女性化乳房
【gainəkoumǽstiə】

Abnormal <u>enlargement</u> of male <u>breasts</u> due to excessive development of the <u>mammary glands</u>.

<u>乳腺</u>の過剰な発達に起因する男性の<u>乳房</u>の異常な<u>肥大</u>.

□ 330
goiter 甲状腺腫
【góitər】

<u>Enlargement</u> of the <u>thyroid gland</u>, commonly visible as a <u>swelling</u> in the anterior[*1] portion of the neck, that is often associated with <u>iodine deficiency</u>.

<u>甲状腺</u>の<u>肥大</u>. 一般に首の前方部分の<u>腫れ</u>として確認でき,しばしば<u>ヨウ素欠乏症</u>と関連する.

[*1] anterior 形 前方の ⇔ posterior 形 後方の

□ 331
hyperglycemia[*1] 高血糖
【haipərglaisí:miə】

Abnormally high <u>concentration</u> of <u>glucose</u> in the <u>circulating blood</u>, seen especially in <u>diabetes mellitus</u>.

循環血液中の異常に高い<u>ブドウ糖</u>の<u>濃度</u>で,主に<u>真性糖尿病</u>にみられる.

[*1] hyperglycemia 名 高血糖 ⇔ hypoglycemia 名 低血糖

□ 332
hyperlipidemia 高脂血症
【haipərlipidí:miə】

Presence of an excessive amount of <u>lipoproteins</u> in the blood.

血中に過剰な量の<u>リポ蛋白</u>が存在すること.

□ 333
hyperuricemia 高尿酸血症
【haipərjùrəsí:miə】

The elevated level of <u>uric acid</u> in <u>blood serum</u> that is above the <u>saturation point</u>.

<u>飽和点</u>を超える<u>血清</u>中の高い<u>尿酸</u>濃度.

症候		定義

□ 334

metabolic acidosis
【mètəbálik æsədóusis】

代謝性アシドーシス

Decreased pH and **bicarbonate** concentration in the **body fluids** caused either by the accumulation of **acids** or by the abnormal loss of **bases** from the body.

酸の蓄積または身体からの塩基の異常喪失により生じる体液のpHおよび重炭酸濃度の減少.

□ 335

metabolic alkalosis
【mètəbálik ælkəlóusis】

代謝性アルカローシス

Abnormally high **alkalinity** of **body fluids** resulting from **hydrogen-ion** loss or excessive intake of alkaline[*1] substances.

水素イオンの喪失またはアルカリ性物質の過剰摂取に起因する体液の異常に高いアルカリ度.

*1 alkaline 形 アルカリ性の ➡ alkalinity 名 アルカリ度

Chapter 14 Vocabulary

Chapter14に収載している医学関連用語の一覧です

英語	日本語	英語	日本語
acid	酸	glucose	ブドウ糖
alkalinity	アルカリ度	growth hormone	成長ホルモン
androgen	アンドロゲン	hydrogen ion	水素イオン
base	塩基	iodine deficiency	ヨウ素欠乏症
bicarbonate	重炭酸	lipoprotein	リポ蛋白
blood serum	血清	mammary gland	乳腺
body fluid	体液	oversecretion	過剰分泌
breast	乳房	pituitary gland	下垂体
circulating blood	循環血液	saturation point	飽和点
concentration	濃度	secondary sex characteristic	二次性徴
diabetes mellitus	真性糖尿病	swelling	腫れ
enlargement	肥大	thyroid gland	甲状腺
epiphyseal line	骨端線	uric acid	尿酸

索 引

英語索引

日本語索引

英語索引

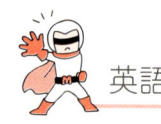

A

abdomen 腹部 …… 16, 73, 78
abdominal cavity 腹腔 …… 32
abdominal distention 腹部膨満 …… 77
abdominal mass 腹部腫瘤 …… 78
abdominal muscle 腹筋 …… 73
abduction 外転 …… 112
abortion 流産 …… 94
abrasion 擦過傷 …… 27, 28
abscess 膿瘍 …… 19
absorption 吸収 …… 74
abulia 無為 …… 101
acalculia 失算 …… 104
acholic stool 無胆汁便 …… 76
acid 酸 …… 120
acne 痤瘡 …… 28
acoustic stimulus 音刺激 …… 45
acquired 後天性の …… 111
acromegaly 末端肥大症 …… 118
activate 活性化する …… 17
activation 活性化 …… 17
acute 急性の …… 27
Adams-Stokes syndrome
　アダムズ・ストークス症候群 …… 64
adaptive behavior 適応行動 …… 98
ADHD 注意欠陥多動性障害 …… 101
Adie syndrome アディー症候群 …… 109
adrenal gland 副腎 …… 84
aggravate 悪化させる …… 53
agnosia 失認 …… 104
agranulocyte 無顆粒白血球 …… 80
agraphia 失書 …… 104
airway 気道 …… 48, 54, 55
airway obstruction 気道閉塞 …… 54
akinesia 無動 …… 104

akinetic 無動の …… 104
akinetic mutism 無動無言症 …… 104
alimentary canal 消化管 …… 74, 78
alkaline アルカリ性の …… 120
alkalinity アルカリ度 …… 120
allergic アレルギーの …… 26
allergic reaction アレルギー反応 …… 26
allergy アレルギー …… 26
alopecia 脱毛症 …… 30
altered consciousness 意識変容 …… 104
alternating pulse 交互脈 …… 63
alveolar 肺胞の …… 56
alveolar ventilation 肺胞換気 …… 56
alveoli（alveolus） 肺胞 …… 50, 54, 56
ambivalence 両価性 …… 100
amenorrhea 無月経 …… 92
amnesia 健忘 …… 97
anal 肛門の …… 76
anal sphincter 肛門括約筋 …… 76
androgen アンドロゲン …… 30, 118
anemia 貧血 …… 81
angioma 血管腫 …… 31
anhidrosis 無汗症 …… 109
ankylosis 関節強直 …… 116
anomaly 異常, 奇形 …… 20
anorexia 食欲不振 …… 73
anterior 前方の …… 119
anterior chamber 前眼房 …… 35, 39
anterior funiculus 前索 …… 113
anterior root 前根 …… 113
anuria 無尿 …… 85
anus 肛門 …… 67, 76, 71
anxiety 不安 …… 99, 102
aorta 大動脈 …… 60, 84
aortic arch 大動脈弓 …… 58

aortic valve 大動脈弁 ……………… 58
aphasia 失語 …………………………… 102
aphtha アフタ ………………………… 29
apnea 無呼吸 ………………… 52, 53, 56
appendix 虫垂 ………………………… 67
appetite 食欲 ………………………… 73
apraxia 失行 ………………………… 103
aqueous flare 房水フレア …………… 39
aqueous humor 眼房水 ……………… 39
Argyll Robertson pupil
　アーガイル・ロバートソン瞳孔 … 109
arm 上腕 ……………………………… 16
aromatic 芳香族の …………………… 70
arrector pili muscle 立毛筋 ………… 22
arrhythmia 不整脈 …………………… 62
arterial 動脈の ……………………… 65
arterial blood 動脈血 ………………… 65
arterial ligament 動脈管索 ………… 58
artery 動脈 ……………………… 22, 65
articulate 発音する ………………… 110
ascending aorta 上行大動脈 ……… 58
ascending colon 上行結腸 ………… 67
ascites 腹水 …………………………… 77
asthenopia 眼精疲労 ………………… 38
ataxia 運動失調 …………………… 114
atrial 心房の ………………………… 59
atrial systole 心房収縮 ……………… 59
atrioventricular block 房室ブロック … 64
atrioventricular valve 房室弁
　………………………… 58, 59, 60, 61
atrium 心房 …………………………… 59
atrophy 萎縮 ………………………… 20
attention 注意 ……………………… 106
attention deficit hyperactivity disorder
　注意欠陥多動性障害 ……………… 101

attention disorder 注意障害 ……… 101
auditory ossicle 耳小骨 ……………… 44
auditory tube 耳管 …………………… 44
auricle 耳介 …………………………… 44
autism 自閉 ………………………… 102
aversion 嫌悪 ………………………… 73

B

Babinski sign バビンスキー徴候 … 112
back 背 ………………………………… 16
bacteria (bacterium) 細菌 ……… 68, 69
base 塩基 …………………………… 120
basophil 好塩基球 …………………… 80
bedsore 床ずれ ……………………… 32
behavioral disorder 行動障害 …… 101
Bell's palsy ベル麻痺 ……………… 109
benign 良性の ………………………… 24
bicarbonate 重炭酸 ………………… 120
bile pigment 胆汁色素 ……………… 76
bilirubin ビリルビン …………… 31, 87
bilirubinuria ビリルビン尿 ………… 87
Biot respiration ビオー呼吸 ………… 53
bipolar cell 双極細胞 ………………… 37
bladder 膀胱 …………… 84, 86, 87, 91, 95
blepharophimosis 瞼裂狭小 ………… 41
blepharoptosis 眼瞼下垂 ……… 41, 109
blind spot 盲斑部 …………………… 35
blindness 失明 ……………………… 40
blood 血液 …………………………… 80
blood flow 血流 ………………… 18, 60, 64
blood level 血中濃度 ………………… 31
blood loss 失血 ……………………… 20
blood pressure 血圧 ……… 64, 104, 115
blood serum 血清 ………………… 119
blood supply 血液供給 ………… 28, 32

英語索引

blood vessel 血管 19
Blumberg sign ブルンベルグ徴候 73
blurred vision かすみ目 38
body fat 体脂肪 18
body fluid 体液 19, 120
body temperature 体温 17
body tissue 体組織 20
borborygmus 腹鳴 77
bowel movement 排便 76
bradycardia 徐脈 62
brain 脳 18
brain dysfunction 脳機能障害 97
brainstem 脳幹 108
breast 乳房 119
breath sound 呼吸音 55
Broca's aphasia ブローカ失語 103
bronchi (bronchus) 気管支 ...50, 51, 53
bronchiole 細気管支 50, 53
bronchospasm 気管支痙攣 53
Brown-Sequard syndrome
　ブラウン・セカール症候群 115
Brudzinski sign ブルジンスキー徴候 ... 110
bulla 水疱 25, 28
burning sensation 灼熱感 71
buttock 殿 16

C

calcification 石灰化 69
calcified 石灰化した 69
calcified tissue 石灰化組織 69
calf ふくらはぎ 64
cancer 癌 32
capillary 毛細血管 23, 27, 31
caput medusae メズサの頭 73
carbon dioxide 二酸化炭素 56

cardia 噴門 75
cardiac 心臓の 60
cardiac arrest 心停止 63
cardiac function 心臓機能 104
cardiac murmur 心雑音 60
cardiopulmonary 心肺の 56
carotid artery (carotid) 頸動脈 62
carotid bruit 頸動脈雑音 62
catatonia 緊張病 101
cecum 盲腸 67
cell 細胞 19, 25
cell fragment 細胞断片 38
cellular 細胞の 25
central fovea 中心窩 35
cerebellum 小脳 108, 114
cerebral 大脳の 64
cerebrum 大脳 64
cerumen 耳垢 46
ceruminous gland 耳道腺 46
cervical 頸部の 109
cervical nerve 頸神経 108
cervical sympathetic chain
　頸部交感神経鎖 109
cervical vertebrae 頸椎 108
cervix 頸部 109
cervix of uterus 子宮頸 90
Chaddock reflex チャドック反射 ... 112
chemical 化学物質 29
chest 胸 16
chest wall 胸壁 55
Cheyne-Stokes respiration
　チェーン・ストークス呼吸 52
childbirth 出産 94
chill 悪寒 17
chorea 舞踏運動 112

choroid 脈絡膜 ……………………… 35
chronic 慢性の ……………………… 27
chyle 乳糜 …………………………… 88
chyluria 乳糜尿 ……………………… 88
ciliary body 毛様体 ………………… 35
ciliary zonule 毛様体小帯 ………… 35
circulating blood 循環血液 ……… 119
circulatory system 循環器系 …… 20, 58
circumscribed 限局性の …………… 24
clinical sign 臨床徴候 …………… 110
clubbed fingers ばち指 …………… 30
coagulate 凝固する ………………… 82
coarse crackle 水泡音 ……………… 54
coccyx 尾骨 ………………………… 108
cochlea 蝸牛 ………………………… 44
cognition 認知 ……………………… 97
cognitive 認知の …………………… 97
cognitive function 認知機能 …… 104, 106
collagen コラーゲン ………………… 28
collecting duct 集合管 …………… 84
color perception 色覚 ……………… 36
coma 昏睡 ………………………… 105
concavity 陥凹 ……………………… 29
concentration 濃度 ……………… 119
conception 受胎 …………………… 93
conductive hearing loss 伝音難聴 … 45
cone 錐体 …………………………… 37
cone cell 錐体細胞 ………………… 37
cone pigment 錐体色素 …………… 36
confabulation 作話 ………………… 97
conflict 葛藤 ……………………… 100
confusion 錯乱 …………………… 106
congenital 先天性の ……………… 20, 111
congestion うっ血 ………………… 23, 77, 78
conjugated bilirubin 抱合型ビリルビン ‥87
conjunctiva 結膜 …………………… 35
consciousness 意識 ……… 64, 97, 105
constipation 便秘 …………………… 76
constriction 縮小 …………………… 40
continuous murmur 連続性雑音 …… 61
contraception 避妊 ………………… 93
contract 収縮する ………………… 18
contraction 収縮
  …………… 18, 40, 48, 53, 70, 74, 112, 113
contralateral 対側の ……………… 115
conversion 転換 ………………… 100
convulsion けいれん ……………… 18, 64
core temperature 核心温度 ……… 17
cornea 角膜 ……………………… 35, 39, 40
corneal 角膜の ……………………… 39
corneal opacity 角膜混濁 ………… 40
cornification 角化 ………………… 27
cornified 角化した ………………… 27
cornified epithelium 角化上皮 …… 33
costa 肋骨 …………………………… 55
costal 肋骨の ……………………… 55
costal pleura 肋骨胸膜 …………… 55
cough 咳 …………………………… 51
cramp 痙攣 ………………………… 64
cramping pain 痙攣痛 ……………… 92
cranial 頭蓋の ……………………… 42
cranial capacity 頭蓋容量 ……… 111
cranial suture 頭蓋縫合 ………… 111
craniosynostosis
  頭蓋縫合早期癒合症 ……………… 111
cranium 頭蓋 …………………… 42, 111
crust 痂皮 ………………………… 28
curvature 彎曲 …………………… 116
cutaneous 皮膚の ………………… 19
cutaneous disorder 皮膚疾患 ……… 30

英語索引

cutis 皮膚 ... 19
cyanosis チアノーゼ ... 65
cyst 囊腫 ... 25
cystocele 膀胱瘤 ... 91

D

day blindness 昼盲症 ... 37
decreased breath sound 呼吸音減弱 ... 55
decubitus 褥瘡 ... 32
defecate 排便する ... 76
defense mechanism 防衛機制 ... 100
deficiency 欠乏 ... 29
dehydration 脱水 ... 19
delayed puberty 思春期遅発症 ... 95
delirium せん妄 ... 106
delusion 妄想 ... 98, 106
delusion of control させられ体験 ... 100
dementia 認知症 ... 97
dental caries う歯 ... 69
depersonalization 離人症 ... 100
deposit 沈着物 ... 28, 68
depression 陥没 ... 48
depressive state うつ状態 ... 99
dermal papilla 真皮乳頭 ... 22
dermis 真皮 ... 22, 26, 27
descending colon 下行結腸 ... 67
desquamated 剥離した ... 68
desquamation 剥離, 落屑 ... 27, 68
developmental disorder 発達障害 ... 101
diabetes 糖尿病 ... 52
diabetes mellitus 真性糖尿病 ... 119
diabetic 糖尿病（性）の ... 52
diabetic ketoacidosis 糖尿病性ケトアシドーシス ... 52

diaphragm 横隔膜 ... 50, 71
diarrhea 下痢 ... 76
diastole 拡張期 ... 59, 61
diastolic 拡張期の ... 59
diastolic blood pressure 拡張期血圧 ... 64
diastolic regurgitant murmur 拡張期逆流性雑音 ... 61
diencephalon 間脳 ... 108
difficulty in breathing 呼吸困難 ... 53
digestive function 消化機能 ... 74
digestive system 消化器系 ... 67
dilate 拡張する ... 23
dilation 拡張 ... 23, 27, 40, 65
dilator muscle 散大筋 ... 40
diplegia 両側麻痺 ... 105
diplopia 複視 ... 38
discharge 排出物 ... 45
discoloration 変色 ... 31, 65
discolored 変色した ... 23
discomfort 不快感 ... 18, 39
disorientation 見当識障害 ... 97, 98
distal 末梢の, 遠位の ... 54
distal airway 末梢気道 ... 54
distention 膨張 ... 72
distractibility 転導性 ... 101
disturbance of consciousness 意識障害 ... 106
disuse 廃用 ... 20
diurnal enuresis 昼間遺尿症 ... 86
dizziness めまい感 ... 115
dorsiflexion 背屈 ... 112
double vision 複視 ... 38
double voiding 二段排尿 ... 87
drug 薬物 ... 30, 33

dry eye　ドライアイ ……………… 39
duodenum　十二指腸 …………… 67, 75
dysarthria　構音障害 ……………… 110
dyschromatopsia　色覚異常 ………… 36
dysfunction　機能不全，機能障害
　…………………………… 19, 70, 109
dysgeusia　味覚異常 ……………… 68
dysmasesis　咀嚼障害 ……………… 70
dysmenorrhea　月経困難 …………… 92
dyspepsia　消化不良 ……………… 74
dysphagia　嚥下障害 …………… 71, 105
dyspnea　呼吸困難 ………………… 56
dystonia　ジストニア ……………… 112
dysuria　排尿痛 …………………… 86

E

ear　耳 ……………………………… 44
earache　耳痛 ……………………… 45
earwax　耳垢 ……………………… 46
edema　浮腫 ……………… 19, 26, 42
egophony　山羊声 ………………… 55
ejaculation　射精 ………………… 95
ejection　駆出 ……………………… 60
elbow　肘 ………………………… 16
elevation　隆起 …………… 24, 25, 26
emaciation　やせ ………………… 18
embryo　胚，胎芽 ……………… 20, 94
embryonic　胚の …………………… 20
embryonic development　胚発生 …… 20
emesis　嘔吐 ……………………… 72
enanthema　粘膜疹 ………………… 29
endbrain　終脳 …………………… 108
endocrine system　内分泌系 ……… 118
enlargement　肥大 … 69, 74, 77, 78, 118, 119
enophthalmos　眼球陥入 ………… 41

environmental stimuli　環境刺激 …… 105
eosinophil　好酸球 ………………… 80
epidermal　表皮の ………………… 27
epidermal cell　表皮細胞 …………… 27
epidermis　表皮 ……………… 22, 27, 26
epididymis　精巣上体 ……………… 90
epidural space　硬膜上腔 ………… 113
epigastric　上腹部の ……………… 74
epigastric pain　上腹部痛 ………… 74
epigastrium　上腹部，心窩部 ……… 74
epiphora　流涙症 ………………… 39
epiphyseal line　骨端線 ………… 118
epistaxis　鼻出血 ………………… 49
epithelium　上皮 ……………… 27, 68
erectile dysfunction　勃起不全 …… 95
erosion　びらん …………………… 26
eructation　おくび ………………… 71
eruption　発疹 …………………… 23, 29
erythema　紅斑 …………………… 23
erythrocyte　赤血球 …………… 80, 81
erythropenia　赤血球減少 ………… 81
esophageal　食道の ……………… 71
esophageal obstruction　食道閉塞 … 71
esophagus　食道 ………… 67, 75, 71
etiology　病因 …………………… 81
excoriation　表皮剥離 …………… 27
excretion　排泄 ………………… 85, 87
exophthalmos　眼球突出 ………… 41
expectorate　喀出する …………… 51
expectoration　喀出 ……………… 51
expiration　呼息，呼気 ……… 48, 53, 54
expiratory　呼息の，呼気の ……… 48
expiratory muscle　呼息筋 ……… 48
exposure　暴露 ………………… 17, 39
extensor muscle　伸筋 ………… 110

英語索引

external acoustic opening　外耳孔 … 44
external auditory canal　外耳道
　……………………………… 44, 45, 46
external ear　外耳 ………………… 44, 45
external genitalia　外陰部 …………… 29
external stimuli　外部刺激 …… 98, 105
external urethral orifice　外尿道口 … 90
extra heart sound　過剰心音 ………… 59
extradural space　硬膜外腔 ………… 113
extremities　四肢 …………………… 114
extremity　末端 ……………………… 30
exudate　滲出物, 滲出液 ……… 25, 52
eye　眼 ………………………………… 35
eye mucus　眼脂 ……………………… 39
eye pain　眼痛 ………………………… 38
eyeball　眼球 …………………… 41, 42
eyelid　眼瞼 …………………………… 35

F

facial muscle　顔面筋 ………… 109, 112
facial nerve　顔面神経 ……………… 109
fascia　筋膜 …………………………… 91
fascial　筋膜の ……………………… 91
fatigue　疲労 ………………………… 38
female genitals　女性器 ……………… 90
fermentation　発酵 …………………… 77
fetor hepaticus　肝性口臭 …………… 70
fetus　胎児 …………………………… 94
fever　発熱 …………………………… 17
fibrous interstitial tissue
　線維性間質組織 …………………… 20
fine crackle　捻髪音 ………………… 54
finger agnosia　手指失認 …………… 104
fissure　亀裂 ………………………… 27
flatus　放屁 …………………………… 71

foot　足 ……………………………… 16
forearm　前腕 ………………………… 16
fourth heart sound　Ⅳ音 …………… 59
friction sound　摩擦音 ……………… 55
frontal lobe　前頭葉 ………………… 108
fundus　胃底 ………………………… 75

G

gallbladder　胆嚢 …………………… 67
gallop rhythm　奔馬調律 …………… 60
ganglion cell　神経(節)細胞 ………… 37
gangrene　壊疽 ……………………… 28
gastric acid　胃酸 …………………… 75
gastric dilatation　胃拡張 …………… 74
gastric juice　胃液 …………………… 71
gastric wall　胃壁 …………………… 74
gastrointestinal tract　胃腸管 ……… 71
gastroptosis　胃下垂 ………………… 74
gastrospasm　胃痙攣 ………………… 74
general condition　全身状態 ………… 16
generalized　全身性の ……………… 29
genitalia　生殖器 …………………… 29
Gerstmann syndrome
　ゲルストマン症候群 …………… 104
gestation　妊娠 ……………………… 94
gigantism　巨人症 …………………… 118
gingiva　歯肉 ………………………… 68
glans penis　陰茎亀頭 ……………… 90
glottis　声門 ………………………… 71
glucose　ブドウ糖 …………… 87, 119
glycosuria　糖尿 ……………………… 87
goiter　甲状腺腫 ……………………… 119
granulocyte　顆粒白血球 …………… 80
gray matter　灰白質 ………………… 113
great toe　拇趾 ……………………… 112

色文字は本書の見出し語です

gross hematuria　肉眼的血尿 ………… 88
growth chart　成長曲線 ………………17
growth hormone　成長ホルモン …… 118
gynecomastia　女性化乳房 …………… 119

H

hair follicle　毛包 ………………… 22, 28
hair loss　脱毛 …………………………30
hair matrix　毛母基 ……………………22
hair papilla　毛乳頭 ……………………22
halitosis　口臭 …………………………70
hallucination　幻覚 ………………98, 106
hand　手 ………………………………16
hard palate　硬口蓋 ……………………68
head　頭 ………………………………16
headache　頭痛 ……………………38, 92
hearing loss　難聴 ……………………45
heart failure　心不全 …………………56
heartbeat　心拍 ……………………62, 63
heartburn　胸やけ …………………71, 74
height　身長 …………………………17
hematemesis　吐血 ……………………75
hematochezia　鮮血便 …………………75
hematologic　血液の，血液学の ……… 78
hematologic disorder　血液疾患 ……… 78
hematology　血液学 ……………………78
hematospermia　血精液症 …………… 91
hematuria　血尿 ………………………88
hemeralopia　昼盲症 …………………37
hemianopia　半盲 ……………………36
hemoglobin　ヘモグロビン ………81, 88
hemoglobinuria　血色素尿 ……………88
hemolysis　溶血 ………………………88
hemopoiesis　造血 ……………………80
hemoptysis　喀血 ………………………51

hemorrhage　出血 ……………………49, 75
hemorrhagic diathesis　出血性素因 … 82
hepatic　肝臓の ………………………70
hepatomegaly　肝腫大 ………………77
hernia　ヘルニア ………………………91
hiccup　しゃっくり ……………………71
hilum　腎門 …………………………84
hip joint　股関節 ……………………110
hives　蕁麻疹 …………………………26
hoarseness　嗄声 ………………………52
hollow viscera　管腔臓器 ……………72
Horner syndrome　ホルネル症候群… 109
hydrogen ion　水素イオン …………120
hyperactivity　多動性 ………………101
hyperchlorhydria　胃酸過多 …………75
hypercoagulable　凝固亢進の ……… 82
hypercoagulable state　凝固亢進状態
　……………………………………………82
hyperemesis gravidarum　妊娠悪阻 … 94
hyperglycemia　高血糖 ……………119
hyperhidrosis　多汗症 ………………30
hyperlipidemia　高脂血症 …………119
hypermenorrhea　月経過多 …………93
hyperphagia　過食症 ………………73
hyperpigmentation　色素沈着過剰 … 32
hypersomnia　過眠 …………………102
hypertension　高血圧 ………………64
hypertrichosis　多毛症 ………………30
hyperuricemia　高尿酸血症 …………119
hyperventilation　過換気 ……………56
hyperviscosity　過粘稠度 ……………82
hypesthesia　感覚鈍麻 …………114, 115
hypochondriasis　心気症 ……………102
hypoglycemia　低血糖 ………………119
hypomenorrhea　月経過少 …………93

索引　英語

英語索引

hyposalivation 唾液分泌不全 68
hypotension 低血圧 64
hypothermia 低体温 17
hypoxemia 低酸素血症 56, 65

I

idiopathic 特発性の 91
ileum 回腸 67
illusion 錯覚 98
immune 免疫の 17
immune disorder 免疫疾患 78
immune system 免疫系 17
immunity 免疫 17
impulse 衝動 98
impulsiveness 衝動性 101
inattentiveness 注意散漫 101
incoordination 協調運動障害 110
induration 硬化 78
infection 感染 28, 32, 40, 78
inferior vena cava 下大静脈 58, 84
infertility 不妊 93
inflammation 炎症 19, 28, 45, 52, 77
inflammatory 炎症性の 28
ingestion 摂取 73
inner ear 内耳 19, 44, 45
innocent murmur 無害性雑音 60
insomnia 不眠 102
inspiration 吸息, 吸気 51, 54, 63
inspiratory 吸息の, 吸気の 51
integument 外皮 22
intercourse 性交 93, 95
intermittent 断続的な 92
intermittent claudication 間欠性跛行
.... 64
internal need 内的欲求 105

interstitial 間質の 20
interstitium 間質 20
interventricular septum 心室中隔 .. 58
intestinal 腸の 77
intestinal gas 腸内ガス 77
intestine 腸 77
intracranial 頭蓋内の 42
intracranial pressure 頭蓋内圧 42
intravascular 血管内の 88
intravascular hemolysis 血管内溶血
.... 88
involuntary 不随意の 18
involuntary movement 不随意運動 ... 112
iodine deficiency ヨウ素欠乏症 119
ipsilateral 同側の 109
iris 虹彩 35, 40
iron deficiency 鉄欠乏 29
irritation 刺激 29, 48, 51
ischemia 虚血 64
itching かゆみ 26, 29

J

jaundice 黄疸 31
jejunum 空腸 67
joint 関節 116
jugular vein 頸静脈 62

K

keloid ケロイド 28
keratosis 角化症 33
Kernig sign ケルニヒ徴候 110
kidney 腎臓 84
Kiesselbach's area
　キーセルバッハ部位 47, 49
knee 膝 16

knee joint　膝関節 ･･････････････････ 110
Korsakoff syndrome
　コルサコフ症候群 ･･････････････････ 97
Kussmaul respiration　クスマウル呼吸
　･････････････････････････････････････ 52
kyphosis　後彎 ･･････････････････････ 116

L

labia majus　大陰唇 ･････････････････ 90
lacrimal　涙の ････････････････････････ 39
lacrimal passage　涙道 ･･････････････ 39
larynx　喉頭 ･･････････････････････ 50, 67
lateral　外側の，側方の ････････････ 112
laxity　弛緩 ･･･････････････････････････ 91
lean body mass　除脂肪体重 ････････ 18
left atrium　左心房 ･･････････････････ 58
left ventricle　左心室 ････････････････ 58
leg　下腿 ･･････････････････････････････ 16
lens　水晶体 ････････････････ 35, 36, 40
lens opacity　水晶体混濁 ･･･････････ 40
lesion　病変 ･･････ 23, 26, 33, 45, 109, 115
leukemia　白血病 ････････････････････ 81
leukemoid reaction　類白血病反応 ･･･ 81
leukocoria　白色瞳孔 ･･･････････････ 40
leukocyte　白血球 ･･･････････ 68, 80, 81
leukocytosis　白血球増加 ･････････････ 81
leukoderma　白斑 ･･･････････････････ 24
leukopenia　白血球減少 ･････････････ 81
leukorrhea　白帯下 ･････････････････ 91
light reflex　対光反射 ･･････････････ 109
limbs　四肢 ･････････････････････････ 112
line　内側を被う ･････････････････････ 51
lingual papillae　舌乳頭 ･････････････ 68
lip　口唇 ･･････････････････････････････ 68
lipoprotein　リポ蛋白 ･････････････ 119

liver　肝臓 ･･････････････････････ 67, 77
lobar bronchi　葉気管支 ･････････････ 50
localized　局在性の ･････････････････ 19
locked-in syndrome　閉じ込め症候群
　･･･････････････････････････････････ 105
lordosis　前彎 ･･････････････････････ 116
lower abdomen　下腹部 ･････････････ 92
lower eyelid　下眼瞼 ････････････････ 41
lower limb　下肢 ････････････････････ 16
lower respiratory tract　下気道 ･････ 50
lumbar　腰部の ････････････････････ 116
lumbar nerve　腰神経 ･･････････････ 108
lumbar vertebrae　腰椎 ････････････ 108
lumen　管腔 ･････････････････････････ 53
lung　肺 ･･･････････････････････ 50, 51, 53
lung tissue　肺組織 ･････････････････ 55
lymph node　リンパ節 ･･･････････････ 32
lymphadenopathy　リンパ節腫脹 ･･････ 32
lymphatic vessel　リンパ管 ･･････････ 88
lymphocyte　リンパ球 ･･･････････････ 80

M

macroglossia　巨大舌 ･･･････････････ 69
macular area　黄斑部 ･･･････････････ 35
macule　斑 ･････････････････････････ 23
malabsorption　吸収不良 ････････････ 74
malaise　倦怠感 ･････････････････････ 18
male genitals　男性器 ･･･････････････ 90
malformation　奇形 ･･････････ 20, 32, 111
malignant　悪性の ･････････････････ 24
malleolus　くるぶし ････････････････ 112
malocclusion　不正咬合 ････････････ 70
mammary gland　乳腺 ････････････ 119
manic state　躁状態 ･････････････････ 99
mass of tissue　組織塊 ･･････････････ 49

英語索引

masseter muscle 咬筋 70
mastication 咀嚼 70
masticatory muscle 咀嚼筋 70
medulla oblongata 延髄 108
megacephaly 大頭症 111
melena 黒色便 76
membrane 膜 25
membranous 膜性の 25
menarche 初経 92
meninges 髄膜 113
meningitis 髄膜炎 110
menopause 閉経 30
menstrual 月経の 92
menstrual cycle 月経周期 92
menstruation 月経 92, 93
mental function 精神機能 97
mental impairment 精神障害 97
mental retardation 精神遅滞 98, 111
metabolic 代謝の 18
metabolic acidosis
　代謝性アシドーシス 52, 120
metabolic alkalosis
　代謝性アルカローシス 120
metabolic disorder 代謝性疾患 77
metabolism 代謝 18, 70, 118
metamorphopsia 変視症 38
meteorism 鼓腸 77
metrorrhagia 不正子宮出血 93
microcephaly 小頭症 111
microscopic hematuria 顕微鏡的血尿 88
midbrain 中脳 108
middiastolic murmur 拡張中期雑音 61
middle ear 中耳 44, 45

midsystolic click 収縮中期クリック 59
miosis 縮瞳 40, 109
mitral valve 僧帽弁 58
mitral valve prolapse 僧帽弁逸脱 59
mittelschmerz 中間痛 92
monocyte 単球 80
mood disorder 気分障害 97
morbid 病的な 102
morning sickness つわり 94
morphologic 形態の, 形態学的な 20
morphologic anomaly 形態異常 20
morphology 形態学 20
motor aphasia 運動性失語 103
motor nerve 運動神経 115
mucosa 粘膜 26
mucous 粘液性の 39
mucous membrane 粘膜
　..... 26, 27, 29, 49, 51, 65, 72
mucus 粘液 39, 51, 91
murmur 雑音 60, 61
muscae volitantes 飛蚊症 38
muscle atrophy 筋萎縮 115
muscle tone 筋緊張 111
muscle weakness 筋力低下 115
muscular defense 筋性防御 73
mydriasis 散瞳 40, 109
myoclonus ミオクローヌス 113
myoglobin ミオグロビン 88
myoglobinuria ミオグロビン尿 88

N

nail 爪 29
nail bed 爪床 30
nape 項 16
nasal bridge 鼻梁 47, 48

nasal cavity 鼻腔 ……… 47, 50, 67, 48	
nasal mucous membrane 鼻粘膜 … 48	
nasal mucus 鼻粘液 ……… 48	
nasal obstruction 鼻閉 ……… 48	
nasal polyp 鼻ポリープ ……… 49	
nausea 悪心 ……… 72, 74, 92, 94	
neck 頸 ……… 16	
necrosis 壊死 ……… 88	
nerve ending 神経終末 ……… 29	
nervous system 神経系 ……… 108	
nervous tissue 神経組織 ……… 115	
neurological 神経の，神経学の … 104	
neurological disorder 神経障害 ……… 104, 105, 109	
neurology 神経学 ……… 104	
neuromuscular disorder 神経筋障害 ……… 71	
neutrophil 好中球 ……… 80	
nevus 母斑 ……… 32	
night blindness 夜盲症 ……… 37	
night sweat 寝汗 ……… 30	
nocturia 夜間頻尿 ……… 85	
nocturnal enuresis 夜尿症 ……… 86	
nodule 結節 ……… 24	
nonviable 成育不可能な ……… 94	
nose 鼻 ……… 47	
nosebleed 鼻出血 ……… 49	
nostril 鼻孔 ……… 47, 50	
nucha 項部 ……… 110	
nuchal 項部の ……… 110	
nuchal rigidity 項部硬直 ……… 110	
numbness しびれ ……… 114	
nutrient 栄養分 ……… 74	
nyctalopia 夜盲症 ……… 37	
nystagmus 眼振 ……… 42

O

obesity 肥満 ……… 18	
obsession 強迫 ……… 98	
obstruction 閉塞 ……… 39, 72, 74, 88	
occipital lobe 後頭葉 ……… 108	
ocular 視覚の，眼の ……… 38	
ocular system 視覚系 ……… 38	
oculus 眼 ……… 38	
olfactory epithelium 嗅上皮 ……… 47	
oligomenorrhea 希発月経 ……… 93	
oliguria 乏尿 ……… 85	
opening snap 開放音 ……… 59	
opposing muscle group 対立筋群 ……… 112	
optic disc 視神経円板 ……… 35, 42	
optic nerve 視神経 ……… 35, 37	
optic papilla 視神経乳頭 ……… 35	
oral bacteria 口内細菌 ……… 70	
oral cavity 口腔 ……… 50, 67, 69	
oral mucosa 口腔粘膜 ……… 29	
orbit 眼窩 ……… 41	
organ 臓器 ……… 20	
organic acid 有機酸 ……… 69	
orthopnea 起坐呼吸 ……… 53	
orthostatic hypotension 起立性低血圧 ……… 115	
oscillation 振動 ……… 42	
otalgia 耳痛 ……… 45	
otogenic 耳原性の ……… 45	
otorrhea 耳漏 ……… 45	
ovary 卵巣 ……… 90, 92	
overgrowth 過形成 ……… 33	
oversecretion 過剰分泌 ……… 118	
ovulation 排卵 ……… 92	
oxygen 酸素 ……… 20

英語索引

oxygen partial pressure　酸素分圧 … 65
oxygenation　酸素化 … 65

P・Q

pain and temperature sensation
　温痛覚 … 115
palatine tonsil　口蓋扁桃 … 68
pallor　蒼白 … 17, 18
palpation　触診 … 55
palpebra　眼瞼 … 41
palpebral　眼瞼の … 41
palpebral fissure　眼瞼裂 … 41
palpitation　動悸 … 63, 99
pancreas　膵臓 … 67
panic attack　パニック発作 … 99
pansystolic murmur　汎収縮期雑音 … 60
papilledema　乳頭浮腫 … 42
papule　丘疹 … 24, 28
paradoxical pulse　奇脈 … 63
paralysis　麻痺 … 109, 110
paranasal sinus　副鼻腔 … 47, 49
paraphasia　錯語 … 103
parasite　寄生虫 … 88
paraumbilical vein　臍傍静脈 … 73
paresthesia　感覚異常 … 114, 115
parietal cell　壁細胞 … 75
parietal lobe　頭頂葉 … 108
Parkinson's disease　パーキンソン病 … 114
parosmia　嗅覚錯誤 … 48
patch　斑 … 23
pelvic　骨盤の … 91
pelvic floor　骨盤底 … 91
pelvis　骨盤 … 91
penile　陰茎の … 95
penis　陰茎 … 90, 95

percentile　パーセンタイル … 17
perception　知覚 … 97
pericardial　心膜の … 61
pericardial friction rub　心膜摩擦音 … 61
pericardium　心膜 … 61
periodic respiration　周期性呼吸 … 52
peripheral　周辺の, 末梢の … 36
peripheral neuropathy　末梢神経障害 … 115
peripheral visual field　周辺視野 … 36
periphery　周辺, 末梢 … 36
peritoneal　腹膜の … 77
peritoneal cavity　腹膜腔 … 77
peritoneum　腹膜 … 77
perspiration　発汗 … 30
pharynx　咽頭 … 50, 67
phobia　恐怖症 … 99
photophobia　羞明 … 39
photopsia　光視症 … 38
photosensitivity　光線過敏症 … 33
physiological　生理的な … 17
physiological response　生理反応 … 17
physiology　生理機能, 生理学 … 17
pigment epithelial cell　色素上皮細胞 … 37
pigmentation　色素沈着 … 24, 32
pituitary gland　下垂体 … 118
plantar　足底の … 112
plantar stimulation　足底刺激 … 112
platelet　血小板 … 80, 82
pleural cavity　胸膜腔 … 52
pleural effusion　胸水 … 52, 55
pleural rub　胸膜摩擦音 … 55
pneumonia　肺炎 … 56
polycythemia　赤血球増加 … 81
polymenorrhea　頻発月経 … 92
polyuria　多尿 … 85

pons 橋	108	pulsus celer 速脈	62
posterior 後方の	119	pulsus paradoxus 奇脈	63
posterior funiculus 後索	113, 114	pulsus tardus 遅脈	63
posterior root 後根	113	pupil 瞳孔	35, 40
precocious puberty 思春期早発症	94	pupillary 瞳孔の	40
pregnancy 妊娠	94	pupillary rigidity 瞳孔強直	109
premature birth 早産	94	purpura 紫斑	23
premature ejaculation 早漏	95	purulence 膿, 化膿	25
primary 原発性の	30	purulent 膿性の, 化膿性の	25
progressive 進行性の	118	purulent matter 膿性物質	51
proliferate 増殖する	24	pus 膿	19, 26, 28
proliferation 増殖	24, 30	pus cell 膿細胞	91
prolonged expiration 呼気延長	53	pustule 膿疱	25, 28
proprioception 固有受容感覚	115	pyloric 幽門の	74
prostate gland 前立腺	90	pyloric area 幽門部	75
protein 蛋白	39	pyloric valve 幽門弁	74
proteinuria 蛋白尿	87	pylorus 幽門	74, 75
protrude 突出する	41	pyramidal tract 錐体路	112
protrusion 突出	41	pyrexia 発熱	17
proximal 近位の	54	pyrosis 胸やけ	71
pruritus 搔痒	29	pyuria 膿尿	88
pseudodementia 仮性認知症	97	quadriplegia 四肢麻痺	105
psychological 心理的な	100		
psychology 心理, 心理学	100	**R**	
psychomotor 精神運動の	101	rash 発疹	23
pubertal 思春期の	94	rebound tenderness 反跳圧痛	73
puberty 思春期	94, 95	recession 陥入	41
pubic 恥骨の	86	rectum 直腸	67
pubis 恥骨	86	red blood cell 赤血球	81
pulmonary 肺の	55	referred pain 関連痛	72
pulmonary artery 肺動脈	58, 60	reflex 反射	73
pulmonary embolism 肺塞栓症	56	reflex movement 反射運動	72
pulmonary pleura 肺胸膜	55	refraction 屈折	36
pulse 脈拍	62, 63, 64	refractive 屈折の	36
pulsus alternans 交互脈	63	refractive error 屈折異常	36

英語索引

regurgitation 逆流 ……………… 71
relaxation 弛緩 ………………… 41
renal artery 腎動脈 …………… 84
renal corpuscle 腎小体 ……… 84
renal cortex 腎皮質 …………… 84
renal medulla 腎髄質 ………… 84
renal pelvis 腎盂 ……………… 84
renal vein 腎静脈 ……………… 84
reproductive system 生殖器系 … 90
respiration 呼吸 ……… 52, 56, 104
respiratory rate 呼吸数 ……… 56
respiratory system 呼吸器系 … 50
respiratory tract 気道 …… 48, 51
retina 網膜 ……………… 35, 36, 40
retrograde ejaculation 逆行性射精 … 95
retropulsion 後方突進 ……… 114
rhinorrhea 鼻漏 ……………… 48
rhonchus いびき様音 ………… 54
right atrium 右心房 …………… 58
right ventricle 右心室 ………… 58
right-left agnosia 左右失認 … 104
rigidity 硬直 ………………… 101
rod 杆体 ……………………… 37
rod cell 杆体細胞 …………… 37
Romberg sign ロンベルク徴候 … 114

S

sac 嚢 ………………………… 25
sacral nerve 仙骨神経 ……… 108
sacrum 仙骨 ………………… 108
saddle nose 鞍鼻 …………… 48
saliva 唾液 …………………… 68
saturation point 飽和点 …… 119
scale 鱗屑 …………………… 27
scar tissue 瘢痕組織 ………… 28

sclera 強膜 …………………… 35
sclerosis 硬化 ………………… 20
scoliosis 側彎 ……………… 116
scotoma 暗点 ………………… 36
scrotum 陰嚢 ………………… 90
sebaceous gland 脂腺 … 22, 28, 31
seborrhea 脂漏 ……………… 31
sebum 皮脂 …………………… 31
secondary sex characteristic
　二次性徴 …………………… 118
secrete 分泌する ……………… 46
secretion 分泌, 分泌物 … 31, 39, 54, 48, 68, 75
self-absorption 自己専心 …… 102
semicircular canal 半規管 …… 44
semilunar valve 半月弁 …… 58, 61
seminal fluid 精液 ………… 91, 95
seminal vesicle 精嚢 ………… 90
sense of smell 嗅覚 ………… 48
sense of taste 味覚 ………… 68
sensitivity 感受性 ……… 68, 114
sensorineural hearing loss 感音難聴 … 45
sensory aphasia 感覚性失語 … 103
sensory nerve 感覚神経 … 29, 115
sensory nerve ending 感覚神経終末 … 29
sensory stimuli 感覚刺激 …… 104
serous 漿液（性）の ………… 19
serous fluid 漿液 …………… 19, 77
serum 漿液 …………………… 19
seventh cranial nerve 第七脳神経 … 109
sexual excitement 性的興奮 … 95
shivering 震え ……………… 17
shock ショック ……………… 20
short stature 低身長 ………… 17
shortness of breath 息切れ … 56, 99
shoulder 肩 …………………… 16

sigmoid colon　S状結腸 …………… 67	stimulation　刺激 ……………………… 38
sign　徴候 ……………………… 94, 95	stimuli (stimulus)　刺激 …… 98, 101, 114
signal node　警報リンパ節 ………… 32	stomach　胃 ……………… 67, 71, 72, 74
skeletal muscle　骨格筋 …………… 18	stool　便 …………………………… 75, 76
skin　皮膚 ………………… 17, 18, 19, 23	strabismus　斜視 …………………… 41
skin furrow　皮溝 …………………… 22	strawberry tongue　イチゴ舌 ……… 68
slough　脱落組織 …………………… 29	stupor　昏迷 …………………… 101, 105
smooth muscle　平滑筋 ………… 53, 74	subarachnoid space　クモ膜下腔 … 113
sneeze　くしゃみ …………………… 48	subcutaneous　皮下の ……………… 19
snore　いびき ………………………… 51	subcutaneous hemorrhage　皮下出血
soft palate　軟口蓋 ………… 50, 68, 51	…………………………………………… 23
solid　充実性の ……………………… 24	subcutaneous tissue　皮下組織 … 19, 22
somatic pain　体性痛 ……………… 72	substernal　胸骨下の ……………… 71
somnolence　傾眠 ………………… 105	sulfur　硫黄 …………………………… 70
spasm　痙攣 ………… 48, 54, 71, 72, 76, 110	sunlight　日光 ………………………… 33
spasmodic　痙攣性の ……………… 48	superficial vein　表在静脈 …………… 65
spasticity　痙縮 ………………… 110, 111	superior vena cava　上大静脈 …… 58
speech muscle　発話筋 …………… 110	supine　仰臥の ……………………… 110
spermatic duct　精管 ……………… 90	supraclavicular fossa　鎖骨上窩 …… 32
sphincter muscle　括約筋 …………… 40	suprapubic　恥骨上の ……………… 86
spider angioma　くも状血管腫 ……… 31	swallowing　嚥下 …………………… 71
spinal arachnoid　脊髄クモ膜 …… 113	sweat　汗 ……………………………… 31
spinal cord　脊髄 ……… 108, 113, 114, 115	sweat gland　汗腺 …………………… 22
spinal dura mater　脊髄硬膜 …… 113	sweating　発汗 …………………… 30, 99
spinal ganglion　脊髄神経節 …… 113	swelling　腫れ ………… 32, 54, 78, 119
spinal pia mater　脊髄軟膜 ……… 113	symptom　症状 …………………… 70, 100
spleen　脾臓 …………………… 67, 78	syncope　失神 ………………… 64, 115
splenomegaly　脾腫 ………………… 78	systemic　全身性の ………………… 30
spoon nail　匙状爪 ………………… 29	systemic disease　全身性疾患 ……… 30
sputum　痰 …………………………… 51	systole　収縮期 ………………… 59, 60, 61
squama　鱗屑 ………………………… 27	systolic blood pressure　収縮期血圧 … 64
starvation　飢餓 …………………… 30	systolic ejection murmur
stenosis　狭窄 …………………… 53, 59	収縮期駆出性雑音 ………………… 60
stenotic　狭窄した ………………… 59	systolic murmur　収縮期雑音 ……… 62
sternum　胸骨 ………………………… 71	systolic pressure　収縮期圧 ………… 63

英語索引

T

tabetic neurosyphilis
　脊髄癆性神経梅毒 109
tachycardia　頻脈 62
tachypnea　頻呼吸 56
tarry stool　タール様便 76
telangiectasia　毛細血管拡張 27
temporal lobe　側頭葉 108
tendon reflex　腱反射 109
tenesmus　しぶり 76
tension　張力 19
testis　精巣 90
tetanus　破傷風 70
tetraplegia　四肢麻痺 105
thigh　大腿 16, 110
third heart sound　Ⅲ音 59
thoracic　胸部の 116
thoracic nerve　胸神経 108
thoracic vertebrae　胸椎 108
thrombocytopenia　血小板減少 82
thrombocytosis　血小板増加 82
thrombus　血栓 82
thyroid gland　甲状腺 119
tingling　刺痛 114
tinnitus　耳鳴り 45
tissue　組織 20, 26, 28, 32, 72
tissue growth　組織増殖 69
tissue loss　組織欠損 26
tongue　舌 68, 69
tongue coating　舌苔 68
tonicity　緊張 112
tooth　歯 68
trachea　気管 50, 51
transudate　漏出液 52
transverse colon　横行結腸 67
transverse myelopathy　横断性脊髄症 115
tremor　振戦 112
tricuspid valve　三尖弁 58
trismus　開口障害 70
trunk　体幹 16
tuberculosis　結核 30
tumor　腫瘍 24, 32, 77
tumor cell　腫瘍細胞 88
turbid　混濁した 39
turbidity　混濁 39
turgor　皮膚緊張度 19
tympanic cavity　鼓室 44
tympanic membrane　鼓膜 44

U

ulcer　潰瘍 26, 29
ulceration　潰瘍化 32
ultraviolet radiation　紫外線 33
umbilicus　臍 73
unconjugated bilirubin
　非抱合型ビリルビン 87
unconsciousness　無意識 105
unilateral　片側の 109
upper eyelid　上眼瞼 41
upper gastrointestinal tract
　上部胃腸管 75
upper limb　上肢 16
upper respiratory tract　上気道 50
ureter　尿管 84
urethra　尿道 84, 86
uric acid　尿酸 119
urinary fistula　尿瘻 87
urinary frequency　頻尿 85
urinary incontinence　尿失禁 86
urinary protein　尿蛋白 87

urinary retention 尿閉 ……… 86
urinary system 泌尿器系 …… 84
urinary tract 尿路 ……… 87
urinary urgency 尿意切迫 …… 86
urination 排尿 ……… 85, 86
urine 尿 ……… 70, 85, 86, 87, 88
urticaria 蕁麻疹 ……… 26
uterine 子宮の ……… 91
uterine bleeding 子宮出血 …… 93
uterine prolapse 子宮脱 ……… 91
uterine tube 卵管 ……… 90
uterus 子宮 ……… 90, 91, 94
uvula 口蓋垂 ……… 68

V

vagina 腟 ……… 90, 91
vaginal orifice 腟口 ……… 90
varicose veins 拡張蛇行静脈 …… 65
vascular 血管の ……… 88
vascular spider くも状血管腫 …… 31
vascularity 血管分布 ……… 32
vegetative state 植物状態 …… 104
vein 静脈 ……… 22
venous hum 静脈こま音 ……… 62
ventricle 心室 ……… 59
ventricular 心室の ……… 59
ventricular filling 心室充満 …… 59
vertebra 脊椎 ……… 113
vertebral column 脊柱 ……… 108, 116
vertigo めまい ……… 19
vesicle 小水疱 ……… 25, 28
vestibular 前庭の ……… 19
vestibular system 前庭系 …… 19
vestibule 前庭 ……… 19, 44
vestibulocochlear nerve 内耳神経 … 44, 45

viable 成育可能な ……… 94
Virchow's node ウィルヒョー結節 …… 32
virilism 男性化 ……… 118
viscera (viscus) 内臓 ……… 72
visceral pain 内臓痛 ……… 72
viscid 粘着性の ……… 91
vision 視力 ……… 36
visual acuity 視力 ……… 37
visual axes (visual axis) 視軸 … 35, 41
visual disturbance 視覚障害 …… 38
visual field 視野 ……… 36
visual field constriction 視野狭窄 ‥ 36
vitreous body 硝子体 ……… 35
vitreous humor 硝子体液 ……… 38
vocal cord 声帯 ……… 50, 52
vocal fremitus 声音震盪 ……… 55
volatile 揮発性の ……… 70
volatile aromatic substance
　揮発性芳香族物質 ……… 70
volatile sulfur compound
　揮発性硫化化合物 ……… 70
voluntary 随意の ……… 18
voluntary movement 随意運動 …… 114
vomit 嘔吐する ……… 72
vomiting 嘔吐 ……… 72, 94

W・X

waist 腰 ……… 16
wakefulness 覚醒 ……… 105
Wernicke's aphasia ウェルニッケ失語 … 103
wheal 膨疹 ……… 26
wheeze 喘鳴 ……… 54
white blood cell 白血球 ……… 81, 88
white matter 白質 ……… 113
xeroderma 乾皮症 ……… 31

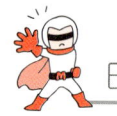

日本語索引

数字

Ⅲ音	third heart sound	59
Ⅳ音	fourth heart sound	59

あ

アーガイル・ロバートソン瞳孔　Argyll Robertson pupil ······ 109
悪性の　malignant ······ 24
足　foot ······ 16
汗　sweat ······ 31
頭　head ······ 16
アダムズ・ストークス症候群　Adams-Stokes syndrome ······ 64
悪化させる　aggravate ······ 53
アディー症候群　Adie syndrome ······ 109
アフタ　aphtha ······ 29
アルカリ性の　alkaline ······ 120
アルカリ度　alkalinity ······ 120
アレルギー　allergy ······ 26
アレルギーの　allergic ······ 26
アレルギー反応　allergic reaction ······ 26
暗点　scotoma ······ 36
アンドロゲン　androgen ······ 30, 118
鞍鼻　saddle nose ······ 48

い

胃　stomach ······ 67, 71, 72, 74
胃液　gastric juice ······ 71
硫黄　sulfur ······ 70
胃拡張　gastric dilatation ······ 74
胃下垂　gastroptosis ······ 74
息切れ　shortness of breath ······ 56, 99
胃痙攣　gastrospasm ······ 74
胃酸　gastric acid ······ 75
胃酸過多　hyperchlorhydria ······ 75
意識　consciousness ······ 64, 97, 105
意識障害　disturbance of consciousness ······ 106
意識変容　altered consciousness ······ 104
萎縮　atrophy ······ 20
異常，奇形　anomaly ······ 20
イチゴ舌　strawberry tongue ······ 68
胃腸管　gastrointestinal tract ······ 71
胃底　fundus ······ 75
いびき　snore ······ 51
いびき様音　rhonchus ······ 54
胃壁　gastric wall ······ 74
陰茎　penis ······ 90, 95
陰茎亀頭　glans penis ······ 90
陰茎の　penile ······ 95
咽頭　pharynx ······ 50, 67
陰嚢　scrotum ······ 90

う

ウィルヒョー結節　Virchow's node ······ 32
ウェルニッケ失語　Wernicke's aphasia ······ 103
う歯　dental caries ······ 69
右心室　right ventricle ······ 58
右心房　right atrium ······ 58
内側を被う　line ······ 51
うっ血　congestion ······ 23, 77, 78
うつ状態　depressive state ······ 99
膿　pus, purulence ······ 19, 25, 26, 28
運動失調　ataxia ······ 114
運動神経　motor nerve ······ 115
運動性失語　motor aphasia ······ 103

え

栄養分　nutrient ······ 74
壊死　necrosis ······ 88
S状結腸　sigmoid colon ······ 67

色文字は本書の見出し語です

壊疽　gangrene　28
遠位の　distal　54
塩基　base　120
嚥下　swallowing　71
嚥下障害　dysphagia　71, 105
炎症　inflammation　19, 28, 45, 52, 77
炎症性の　inflammatory　28
延髄　medulla oblongata　108

お

横隔膜　diaphragm　50, 71
横行結腸　transverse colon　67
黄疸　jaundice　31
横断性脊髄症　transverse myelopathy　115
嘔吐　emesis, vomiting　72, 94
嘔吐する　vomit　72
黄斑部　macular area　35
悪寒　chill　17
おくび　eructation　71
悪心　nausea　72, 74, 92, 94
音刺激　acoustic stimulus　45
温痛覚　pain and temperature sensation　115

か

外陰部　external genitalia　29
開口障害　trismus　70
外耳　external ear　44, 45
外耳孔　external acoustic opening　44
外耳道　external auditory canal　44, 45, 46
外側の　lateral　112
回腸　ileum　67
外転　abduction　112
外尿道口　external urethral orifice　90
灰白質　gray matter　113
外皮　integument　22

外部刺激　external stimuli　98, 105
開放音　opening snap　59
潰瘍　ulcer　26, 29
潰瘍化　ulceration　32
化学物質　chemical　29
過換気　hyperventilation　56
下眼瞼　lower eyelid　41
下気道　lower respiratory tract　50
蝸牛　cochlea　44
角化　cornification　27
角化した　cornified　27
角化症　keratosis　33
角化上皮　cornified epithelium　33
喀出　expectoration　51
喀出する　expectorate　51
核心温度　core temperature　17
覚醒　wakefulness　105
拡張　dilation　23, 27, 40, 65
拡張期　diastole　59, 61
拡張期逆流性雑音
　diastolic regurgitant murmur　61
拡張期血圧　diastolic blood pressure　64
拡張期の　diastolic　59
拡張する　dilate　23
拡張蛇行静脈　varicose veins　65
拡張中期雑音　middiastolic murmur　61
角膜　cornea　35, 39, 40
角膜混濁　corneal opacity　40
角膜の　corneal　39
過形成　overgrowth　33
下行結腸　descending colon　67
下肢　lower limb　16
過剰心音　extra heart sound　59
過剰分泌　oversecretion　118
過食症　hyperphagia　73

日本語索引

下垂体 pituitary gland	118
かすみ目 blurred vision	38
仮性認知症 pseudodementia	97
肩 shoulder	16
下腿 leg	16
下大静脈 inferior vena cava	58, 84
喀血 hemoptysis	51
活性化 activation	17
活性化する activate	17
葛藤 conflict	100
括約筋 sphincter muscle	40
過粘稠度 hyperviscosity	82
化膿 purulence	25
化膿性の purulent	25
痂皮 crust	28
下腹部 lower abdomen	92
過眠 hypersomnia	102
かゆみ itching	26, 29
顆粒白血球 granulocyte	80
癌 cancer	32
陥凹 concavity	29
感音難聴 sensorineural hearing loss	45
眼窩 orbit	41
感覚異常 paresthesia	114, 115
感覚刺激 sensory stimuli	104
感覚神経 sensory nerve	29, 115
感覚神経終末 sensory nerve ending	29
感覚性失語 sensory aphasia	103
感覚鈍麻 hypesthesia	114, 115
眼球 eyeball	41, 42
眼球陥入 enophthalmos	41
眼球突出 exophthalmos	41
環境刺激 environmental stimuli	105
管腔 lumen	53
管腔臓器 hollow viscera	72
間欠性跛行 intermittent claudication	64
眼瞼 palpebra, eyelid	35, 41
眼瞼下垂 blepharoptosis	41, 109
眼瞼の palpebral	41
眼瞼裂 palpebral fissure	41
眼脂 eye mucus	39
間質 interstitium	20
間質の interstitial	20
感受性 sensitivity	68, 114
肝腫大 hepatomegaly	77
眼振 nystagmus	42
肝性口臭 fetor hepaticus	70
眼精疲労 asthenopia	38
関節 joint	116
関節強直 ankylosis	116
汗腺 sweat gland	22
感染 infection	28, 32, 40, 78
肝臓 liver	67, 77
肝臓の hepatic	70
杆体 rod	37
杆体細胞 rod cell	37
眼痛 eye pain	38
陥入 recession	41
間脳 diencephalon	108
乾皮症 xeroderma	31
眼房水 aqueous humor	39
陥没 depression	48
顔面筋 facial muscle	109, 112
顔面神経 facial nerve	109
関連痛 referred pain	72

き

キーセルバッハ部位 Kiesselbach's area	47, 49
飢餓 starvation	30
気管 trachea	50, 51

気管支　bronchi（bronchus）……50, 51, 53
気管支痙攣　bronchospasm……………53
奇形　malformation……………20, 32, 111
起坐呼吸　orthopnea………………………53
寄生虫　parasite………………………………88
気道　respiratory tract, airway ‥48, 51, 54, 55
気道閉塞　airway obstruction …………54
機能障害　dysfunction ………………… 109
機能不全　dysfunction ……………… 19, 70
希発月経　oligomenorrhea ………………93
揮発性の　volatile…………………………70
揮発性芳香族物質
　　volatile aromatic substance …………70
揮発性硫化化合物　volatile sulfur compound‥70
気分障害　mood disorder ………………97
奇脈
　　paradoxical pulse, pulsus paradoxus…63
逆流　regurgitation ………………………71
逆行性射精　retrograde ejaculation ……95
嗅覚　sense of smell………………………48
嗅覚錯誤　parosmia………………………48
吸気　inspiration………………51, 54, 63
吸気の　inspiratory………………………51
吸収　absorption……………………………74
吸収不良　malabsorption …………………74
嗅上皮　olfactory epithelium …………47
丘疹　papule ……………………………24, 28
急性の　acute ………………………………27
吸息　inspiration………………51, 54, 63
吸息の　inspiratory………………………51
橋　pons ………………………………… 108
仰臥の　supine ………………………… 110
凝固亢進状態　hypercoagulable state ‥82
凝固亢進の　hypercoagulable …………82
凝固する　coagulate………………………82

胸骨　sternum ……………………………71
胸骨下の　substernal ……………………71
狭窄　stenosis ………………………… 53, 59
狭窄した　stenotic ………………………59
胸神経　thoracic nerve………………… 108
胸水　pleural effusion………………52, 55
協調運動障害　incoordination ………… 110
胸椎　thoracic vertebrae……………… 108
強迫　obsession……………………………98
恐怖症　phobia ……………………………99
胸部の　thoracic ……………………… 116
胸壁　chest wall……………………………55
強膜　sclera…………………………………35
胸膜腔　pleural cavity……………………52
胸膜摩擦音　pleural rub…………………55
局在性の　localized ………………………19
虚血　ischemia ……………………………64
巨人症　gigantism……………………… 118
巨大舌　macroglossia ……………………69
起立性低血圧　orthostatic hypotension … 115
亀裂　fissure…………………………………27
筋萎縮　muscle atrophy……………… 115
近位の　proximal …………………………54
筋緊張　muscle tone ………………… 111
筋性防御　muscular defense……………73
緊張　tonicity……………………………… 112
緊張病　catatonia……………………… 101
筋膜　fascia…………………………………91
筋膜の　fascial ……………………………91
筋力低下　muscle weakness………… 115

く

空腸　jejunum ………………………………67
くしゃみ　sneeze …………………………48
駆出　ejection………………………………60

日本語索引

クスマウル呼吸 Kussmaul respiration……52
屈折 refraction……36
屈折異常 refractive error……36
屈折の refractive……36
くも状血管腫
    vascular spider, spider angioma……31
クモ膜下腔 subarachnoid space……113
くるぶし malleolus……112

け

頸 neck……16
痙縮 spasticity……110, 111
頸静脈 jugular vein……62
頸神経 cervical nerve……108
形態異常 morphologic anomaly……20
形態学 morphology……20
形態学的な morphologic……20
形態の morphologic……20
頸椎 cervical vertebrae……108
頸動脈 carotid artery (carotid)……62
頸動脈雑音 carotid bruit……62
頸部 cervix……109
頸部交感神経鎖
    cervical sympathetic chain……109
頸部の cervical……109
警報リンパ節 signal node……32
傾眠 somnolence……105
けいれん(全身性のもの) convulsion……18, 64
痙攣（局所性のもの） cramp, spasm
    ……48, 54, 64, 71, 72, 76, 110
痙攣性の spasmodic……48
痙攣痛 cramping pain……92
血圧 blood pressure……64, 104, 115
血液 blood……80
血液学 hematology……78
血液学の hematologic……78
血液供給 blood supply……28, 32
血液疾患 hematologic disorder……78
血液の hematologic……78
結核 tuberculosis……30
血管 blood vessel……19
血管腫 angioma……31
血管内の intravascular……88
血管内溶血 intravascular hemolysis……88
血管の vascular……88
血管分布 vascularity……32
月経 menstruation……92, 93
月経過少 hypomenorrhea……93
月経過多 hypermenorrhea……93
月経困難 dysmenorrhea……92
月経周期 menstrual cycle……92
月経の menstrual……92
血色素尿 hemoglobinuria……88
血小板 platelet……80, 82
血小板減少 thrombocytopenia……82
血小板増加 thrombocytosis……82
血清 blood serum……119
血精液症 hematospermia……91
結節 nodule……24
血栓 thrombus……82
血中濃度 blood level……31
血尿 hematuria……88
欠乏 deficiency……29
結膜 conjunctiva……35
血流 blood flow……18, 60, 64
下痢 diarrhea……76
ゲルストマン症候群 Gerstmann syndrome……104
ケルニヒ徴候 Kernig sign……110
ケロイド keloid……28
嫌悪 aversion……73

日本語	英語	ページ
幻覚	hallucination	98, 106
限局性の	circumscribed	24
倦怠感	malaise	18
見当識障害	disorientation	97, 98
原発性の	primary	30
腱反射	tendon reflex	109
顕微鏡的血尿	microscopic hematuria	88
健忘	amnesia	97
瞼裂狭小	blepharophimosis	41

こ

日本語	英語	ページ
項	nape	16
好塩基球	basophil	80
構音障害	dysarthria	110
硬化	sclerosis, induration	20, 78
口蓋垂	uvula	68
口蓋扁桃	palatine tonsil	68
咬筋	masseter muscle	70
口腔	oral cavity	50, 67, 69
口腔粘膜	oral mucosa	29
高血圧	hypertension	64
高血糖	hyperglycemia	119
硬口蓋	hard palate	68
交互脈	alternating pulse, pulsus alternans	63
後根	posterior root	113
虹彩	iris	35, 40
後索	posterior funiculus	113, 114
好酸球	eosinophil	80
高脂血症	hyperlipidemia	119
光視症	photopsia	38
口臭	halitosis	70
甲状腺	thyroid gland	119
甲状腺腫	goiter	119
口唇	lip	68
光線過敏症	photosensitivity	33
好中球	neutrophil	80
硬直	rigidity	101
後天性の	acquired	111
喉頭	larynx	50, 67
行動障害	behavioral disorder	101
後頭葉	occipital lobe	108
口内細菌	oral bacteria	70
高尿酸血症	hyperuricemia	119
紅斑	erythema	23
項部	nucha	110
項部硬直	nuchal rigidity	110
項部の	nuchal	110
後方突進	retropulsion	114
後方の	posterior	119
硬膜外腔	extradural space	113
硬膜上腔	epidural space	113
肛門	anus	67, 76, 71
肛門括約筋	anal sphincter	76
肛門の	anal	76
後彎	kyphosis	116
股関節	hip joint	110
呼気	expiration	48, 53, 54
呼気延長	prolonged expiration	53
呼気の	expiratory	48
呼吸	respiration	52, 56, 104
呼吸音	breath sound	55
呼吸音減弱	decreased breath sound	55
呼吸器系	respiratory system	50
呼吸困難	difficulty in breathing, dyspnea	53, 56
呼吸数	respiratory rate	56
黒色便	melena	76
腰	waist	16
鼓室	tympanic cavity	44
呼息	expiration	48, 53, 54

日本語索引

日本語	英語	ページ
呼息筋	expiratory muscle	48
呼息の	expiratory	48
鼓腸	meteorism	77
骨格筋	skeletal muscle	18
骨端線	epiphyseal line	118
骨盤	pelvis	91
骨盤底	pelvic floor	91
骨盤の	pelvic	91
鼓膜	tympanic membrane	44
固有受容感覚	proprioception	115
コラーゲン	collagen	28
コルサコフ症候群	Korsakoff syndrome	97
昏睡	coma	105
混濁	turbidity	39
混濁した	turbid	39
昏迷	stupor	101, 105

さ

日本語	英語	ページ
臍	umbilicus	73
細気管支	bronchiole	50, 53
細菌	bacteria (bacterium)	68, 69
細胞	cell	19, 25
臍傍静脈	paraumbilical vein	73
細胞断片	cell fragment	38
細胞の	cellular	25
錯語	paraphasia	103
錯乱	confusion	106
作話	confabulation	97
鎖骨上窩	supraclavicular fossa	32
匙状爪	spoon nail	29
左心室	left ventricle	58
左心房	left atrium	58
嗄声	hoarseness	52
させられ体験	delusion of control	100
痤瘡	acne	28
雑音	murmur	60, 61
錯覚	illusion	98
擦過傷	abrasion	27, 28
左右失認	right-left agnosia	104
酸	acid	120
三尖弁	tricuspid valve	58
酸素	oxygen	20
酸素化	oxygenation	65
酸素分圧	oxygen partial pressure	65
散大筋	dilator muscle	40
散瞳	mydriasis	40, 109

し

日本語	英語	ページ
耳介	auricle	44
紫外線	ultraviolet radiation	33
視覚系	ocular system	38
視覚障害	visual disturbance	38
視覚の	ocular	38
弛緩	relaxation, laxity	41, 91
耳管	auditory tube	44
色覚	color perception	36
色覚異常	dyschromatopsia	36
色素上皮細胞	pigment epithelial cell	37
色素沈着	pigmentation	24, 32
色素沈着過剰	hyperpigmentation	32
子宮	uterus	90, 91, 94
子宮頸	cervix of uterus	90
子宮出血	uterine bleeding	93
子宮脱	uterine prolapse	91
子宮の	uterine	91
刺激	irritation, stimulation, stimuli (stimulus)	29, 38, 48, 51, 98, 101, 114
耳原性の	otogenic	45
耳垢	cerumen, earwax	46
自己専心	self-absorption	102

四肢	limbs, extremities ············· 112, 114
視軸	visual axes（visual axis）······· 35, 41
四肢麻痺	tetraplegia, quadriplegia ··· 105
思春期	puberty ······························ 94, 95
思春期早発症	precocious puberty ······· 94
思春期遅発症	delayed puberty ············· 95
思春期の	pubertal ··································· 94
耳小骨	auditory ossicle ························· 44
視神経	optic nerve ························ 35, 37
視神経円板	optic disc ······················ 35, 42
視神経乳頭	optic papilla ························ 35
ジストニア	dystonia ···························· 112
脂腺	sebaceous gland ············· 22, 28, 31
刺痛	tingling ··································· 114
耳痛	otalgia, earache ························ 45
膝関節	knee joint ······························ 110
失血	blood loss ································ 20
失語	aphasia ································· 102
失行	apraxia ································· 103
失算	acalculia ······························· 104
失書	agraphia ······························· 104
失神	syncope ··························· 64, 115
失認	agnosia ································· 104
失明	blindness ································· 40
耳道腺	ceruminous gland ···················· 46
歯肉	gingiva ···································· 68
紫斑	purpura ···································· 23
しびれ	numbness ···························· 114
しぶり	tenesmus ······························ 76
自閉	autism ··································· 102
視野	visual field ····························· 36
視野狭窄	visual field constriction ······· 36
灼熱感	burning sensation ···················· 71
斜視	strabismus ······························ 41
射精	ejaculation ······························ 95

しゃっくり	hiccup ······························ 71
周期性呼吸	periodic respiration ········· 52
集合管	collecting duct ························ 84
充実性の	solid ···································· 24
収縮	contraction ·· 18, 40, 48, 53, 70, 74, 112, 113
収縮期	systole ······················· 59, 60, 61
収縮期圧	systolic pressure ···················· 63
収縮期駆出性雑音	
	systolic ejection murmur ······· 60
収縮期血圧	systolic blood pressure ······· 64
収縮期雑音	systolic murmur ················ 62
収縮する	contract ································ 18
収縮中期クリック	midsystolic click ······ 59
重炭酸	bicarbonate ·························· 120
十二指腸	duodenum ························ 67, 75
終脳	endbrain ································ 108
周辺	periphery ································ 36
周辺視野	peripheral visual field ·········· 36
周辺の	peripheral ······························ 36
羞明	photophobia ···························· 39
縮小	constriction ····························· 40
縮瞳	miosis ······························ 40, 109
手指失認	finger agnosia ······················ 104
受胎	conception ······························ 93
出血	hemorrhage ······················ 49, 75
出血性素因	hemorrhagic diathesis ····· 82
出産	childbirth ································ 94
腫瘍	tumor ······························ 24, 32, 77
腫瘍細胞	tumor cell ····························· 88
循環器系	circulatory system ··········· 20, 58
循環血液	circulating blood ··············· 119
漿液	serum, serous fluid ············· 19, 77
漿液（性）の	serous ································ 19
消化管	alimentary canal ··················· 74, 78
消化器系	digestive system ··················· 67

日本語索引

消化機能　digestive function ……… 74
消化不良　dyspepsia ……… 74
上眼瞼　upper eyelid ……… 41
上気道　upper respiratory tract ……… 50
上行結腸　ascending colon ……… 67
上行大動脈　ascending aorta ……… 58
上肢　upper limb ……… 16
硝子体　vitreous body ……… 35
硝子体液　vitreous humor ……… 38
症状　symptom ……… 70, 100
小水疱　vesicle ……… 25, 28
上大静脈　superior vena cava ……… 58
衝動　impulse ……… 98
小頭症　microcephaly ……… 111
衝動性　impulsiveness ……… 101
小脳　cerebellum ……… 108, 114
上皮　epithelium ……… 27, 68
上部胃腸管　upper gastrointestinal tract ……… 75
上腹部　epigastrium ……… 74
上腹部痛　epigastric pain ……… 74
上腹部の　epigastric ……… 74
静脈　vein ……… 22
静脈こま音　venous hum ……… 62
上腕　arm ……… 16
触診　palpation ……… 55
褥瘡　decubitus ……… 32
食道　esophagus ……… 67, 75, 71
食道の　esophageal ……… 71
食道閉塞　esophageal obstruction ……… 71
植物状態　vegetative state ……… 104
食欲　appetite ……… 73
食欲不振　anorexia ……… 73
初経　menarche ……… 92
除脂肪体重　lean body mass ……… 18
女性化乳房　gynecomastia ……… 119

女性器　female genitals ……… 90
ショック　shock ……… 20
徐脈　bradycardia ……… 62
視力　vision, visual acuity ……… 36, 37
脂漏　seborrhea ……… 31
耳漏　otorrhea ……… 45
心窩部　epigastrium ……… 74
腎盂　renal pelvis ……… 84
心気症　hypochondriasis ……… 102
伸筋　extensor muscle ……… 110
神経学　neurology ……… 104
神経学の　neurological ……… 104
神経筋障害　neuromuscular disorder ……… 71
神経系　nervous system ……… 108
神経終末　nerve ending ……… 29
神経障害　neurological disorder ……… 104, 105, 109
神経(節)細胞　ganglion cell ……… 37
神経組織　nervous tissue ……… 115
神経の　neurological ……… 104
進行性の　progressive ……… 118
心雑音　cardiac murmur ……… 60
心室　ventricle ……… 59
心室充満　ventricular filling ……… 59
心室中隔　interventricular septum ……… 58
心室の　ventricular ……… 59
滲出液　exudate ……… 52
滲出物　exudate ……… 25
腎小体　renal corpuscle ……… 84
腎静脈　renal vein ……… 84
腎髄質　renal medulla ……… 84
真性糖尿病　diabetes mellitus ……… 119
振戦　tremor ……… 112
腎臓　kidney ……… 84
心臓機能　cardiac function ……… 104
心臓の　cardiac ……… 60

日本語	英語	ページ
身長	height	17
心停止	cardiac arrest	63
振動	oscillation	42
腎動脈	renal artery	84
心肺の	cardiopulmonary	56
心拍	heartbeat	62, 63
真皮	dermis	22, 26, 27
腎皮質	renal cortex	84
真皮乳頭	dermal papilla	22
心不全	heart failure	56
心房	atrium	59
心房収縮	atrial systole	59
心房の	atrial	59
心膜	pericardium	61
心膜の	pericardial	61
心膜摩擦音	pericardial friction rub	61
蕁麻疹	urticaria, hives	26
腎門	hilum	84
心理	psychology	100
心理学	psychology	100
心理的な	psychological	100

す

随意運動	voluntary movement	114
随意の	voluntary	18
水晶体	lens	35, 36, 40
水晶体混濁	lens opacity	40
水素イオン	hydrogen ion	120
膵臓	pancreas	67
錐体	cone	37
錐体細胞	cone cell	37
錐体色素	cone pigment	36
錐体路	pyramidal tract	112
水疱	bulla	25, 28
水泡音	coarse crackle	54

髄膜	meninges	113
髄膜炎	meningitis	110
頭痛	headache	38, 92

せ

背	back	16
成育可能な	viable	94
成育不可能な	nonviable	94
精液	seminal fluid	91, 95
声音震盪	vocal fremitus	55
精管	spermatic duct	90
性交	intercourse	93, 95
生殖器	genitalia	29
生殖器系	reproductive system	90
精神運動の	psychomotor	101
精神機能	mental function	97
精神障害	mental impairment	97
精神遅滞	mental retardation	98, 111
精巣	testis	90
精巣上体	epididymis	90
声帯	vocal cord	50, 52
成長曲線	growth chart	17
成長ホルモン	growth hormone	118
性的興奮	sexual excitement	95
精嚢	seminal vesicle	90
声門	glottis	71
生理学	physiology	17
生理機能	physiology	17
生理的な	physiological	17
生理反応	physiological response	17
咳	cough	51
脊髄	spinal cord	108, 113, 114, 115
脊髄クモ膜	spinal arachnoid	113
脊髄硬膜	spinal dura mater	113
脊髄神経節	spinal ganglion	113

日本語索引

脊髄軟膜　spinal pia mater ……… 113
脊髄癆性神経梅毒　tabetic neurosyphilis … 109
脊柱　vertebral column…………… 108, 116
脊椎　vertebra ……………………… 113
舌　tongue………………………… 68, 69
石灰化　calcification ……………… 69
石灰化した　calcified …………… 69
石灰化組織　calcified tissue …… 69
赤血球　erythrocyte, red blood cell ‥ 80, 81
赤血球減少　erythropenia ……… 81
赤血球増加　polycythemia……… 81
摂取　ingestion …………………… 73
舌苔　tongue coating…………… 68
舌乳頭　lingual papillae ………… 68
線維性間質組織　fibrous interstitial tissue ‥ 20
前眼房　anterior chamber ……… 35, 39
鮮血便　hematochezia…………… 75
仙骨　sacrum ……………………… 108
仙骨神経　sacral nerve ………… 108
前根　anterior root ……………… 113
前索　anterior funiculus………… 113
全身状態　general condition …… 16
全身性疾患　systemic disease … 30
全身性の　generalized, systemic…… 29, 30
前庭　vestibule…………………… 19, 44
前庭系　vestibular system ……… 19
前庭の　vestibular ……………… 19
先天性の　congenital…………… 20, 111
前頭葉　frontal lobe ……………… 108
前方の　anterior ………………… 119
喘鳴　wheeze …………………… 54
せん妄　delirium………………… 106
前立腺　prostate gland ………… 90
前腕　forearm …………………… 16
前彎　lordosis …………………… 116

そ

臓器　organ ……………………… 20
双極細胞　bipolar cell…………… 37
造血　hemopoiesis ……………… 80
早産　premature birth …………… 94
爪床　nail bed …………………… 30
躁状態　manic state……………… 99
増殖　proliferation……………… 24, 30
増殖する　proliferate …………… 24
蒼白　pallor ……………………… 17, 18
僧帽弁　mitral valve……………… 58
僧帽弁逸脱　mitral valve prolapse……… 59
掻痒　pruritus …………………… 29
早漏　premature ejaculation …… 95
足底刺激　plantar stimulation ……… 112
足底の　plantar ………………… 112
側頭葉　temporal lobe…………… 108
側方の　lateral ………………… 112
速脈　pulsus celer ……………… 62
側彎　scoliosis …………………… 116
組織　tissue ……………………… 20, 26, 28, 32, 72
組織塊　mass of tissue ………… 49
組織欠損　tissue loss…………… 26
組織増殖　tissue growth ……… 69
咀嚼　mastication ……………… 70
咀嚼筋　masticatory muscle…… 70
咀嚼障害　dysmasesis…………… 70

た

タール様便　tarry stool ………… 76
大陰唇　labia majus……………… 90
体液　body fluid ………………… 19, 120
体温　body temperature ………… 17
胎芽　embryo …………………… 94
体幹　trunk ……………………… 16

色文字は本書の見出し語です

対光反射　light reflex ……………………… 109
胎児　fetus ……………………………………… 94
体脂肪　body fat ………………………………… 18
代謝　metabolism …………………… 18, 70, 118
代謝性アシドーシス　metabolic acidosis
　………………………………………………… 52, 120
代謝性アルカローシス　metabolic alkalosis ‥ 120
代謝性疾患　metabolic disorder ………… 77
代謝の　metabolic ……………………………… 18
体性痛　somatic pain ………………………… 72
対側の　contralateral ……………………… 115
体組織　body tissue …………………………… 20
大腿　thigh ……………………………… 16, 110
大頭症　megacephaly …………………… 111
大動脈　aorta …………………………… 60, 84
大動脈弓　aortic arch ………………………… 58
大動脈弁　aortic valve ………………………… 58
第七脳神経　seventh cranial nerve … 109
大脳　cerebrum ………………………………… 64
大脳の　cerebral ……………………………… 64
対立筋群　opposing muscle group … 112
唾液　saliva ……………………………………… 68
唾液分泌不全　hyposalivation ……………… 68
多汗症　hyperhidrosis ………………………… 30
脱水　dehydration …………………………… 19
脱毛　hair loss ………………………………… 30
脱毛症　alopecia ……………………………… 30
脱落組織　slough ……………………………… 29
多動性　hyperactivity ……………………… 101
多尿　polyuria ………………………………… 85
多毛症　hypertrichosis ……………………… 30
痰　sputum ……………………………………… 51
単球　monocyte ………………………………… 80
胆汁色素　bile pigment ……………………… 76
男性化　virilism ……………………………… 118

男性器　male genitals ………………………… 90
断続的な　intermittent ……………………… 92
胆嚢　gallbladder ……………………………… 67
蛋白　protein …………………………………… 39
蛋白尿　proteinuria ………………………… 87

ち

チアノーゼ　cyanosis ………………………… 65
チェーン・ストークス呼吸
　　Cheyne-Stokes respiration ………… 52
知覚　perception ……………………………… 97
恥骨　pubis ……………………………………… 86
恥骨上の　suprapubic ………………………… 86
恥骨の　pubic …………………………………… 86
腟　vagina ……………………………… 90, 91
腟口　vaginal orifice …………………………… 90
遅脈　pulsus tardus ………………………… 63
チャドック反射　Chaddock reflex …… 112
注意　attention ……………………………… 106
注意欠陥多動性障害　attention deficit
　　hyperactivity disorder（ADHD）… 101
注意散漫　inattentiveness ………………… 101
注意障害　attention disorder …………… 101
昼間遺尿症　diurnal enuresis …………… 86
中間痛　mittelschmerz ……………………… 92
中耳　middle ear ……………………… 44, 45
中心窩　central fovea ………………………… 35
虫垂　appendix ………………………………… 67
中脳　midbrain ……………………………… 108
昼盲症　hemeralopia, day blindness …… 37
腸　intestine …………………………………… 77
徴候　sign …………………………… 94, 95
腸内ガス　intestinal gas …………………… 77
腸の　intestinal ………………………………… 77
張力　tension …………………………………… 19

日本語索引

直腸　rectum 67
沈着物　deposit 28, 68

つ・て

爪　nail 29
つわり　morning sickness 94
手　hand 16
低血圧　hypotension 64
低血糖　hypoglycemia 119
低酸素血症　hypoxemia 56, 65
低身長　short stature 17
低体温　hypothermia 17
適応行動　adaptive behavior 98
鉄欠乏　iron deficiency 29
殿　buttock 16
伝音難聴　conductive hearing loss 45
転換　conversion 100
転導性　distractibility 101

と

頭蓋　cranium 42, 111
頭蓋内圧　intracranial pressure 42
頭蓋内の　intracranial 42
頭蓋の　cranial 42
頭蓋縫合　cranial suture 111
頭蓋縫合早期癒合症　craniosynostosis ... 111
頭蓋容量　cranial capacity 111
動悸　palpitation 63, 99
瞳孔　pupil 35, 40
瞳孔強直　pupillary rigidity 109
瞳孔の　pupillary 40
同側の　ipsilateral 109
頭頂葉　parietal lobe 108
糖尿　glycosuria 87
糖尿病　diabetes 52

糖尿病性ケトアシドーシス
　　diabetic ketoacidosis 52
糖尿病（性）の　diabetic 52
動脈　artery 22, 65
動脈管索　arterial ligament 58
動脈血　arterial blood 65
動脈の　arterial 65
特発性の　idiopathic 91
吐血　hematemesis 75
床ずれ　bedsore 32
閉じ込め症候群　locked-in syndrome ... 105
突出　protrusion 41
突出する　protrude 41
ドライアイ　dry eye 39

な

内耳　inner ear 19, 44, 45
内耳神経　vestibulocochlear nerve .. 44, 45
内臓　viscera (viscus) 72
内臓痛　visceral pain 72
内的欲求　internal need 105
内分泌系　endocrine system 118
涙の　lacrimal 39
軟口蓋　soft palate 50, 68, 51
難聴　hearing loss 45

に

肉眼的血尿　gross hematuria 88
二酸化炭素　carbon dioxide 56
二次性徴　secondary sex characteristic
　　.. 118
二段排尿　double voiding 87
日光　sunlight 33
乳腺　mammary gland 119
乳頭浮腫　papilledema 42

乳糜 chyle	88
乳糜尿 chyluria	88
乳房 breast	119
尿 urine	70, 85, 86, 87, 88
尿意切迫 urinary urgency	86
尿管 ureter	84
尿酸 uric acid	119
尿失禁 urinary incontinence	86
尿蛋白 urinary protein	87
尿道 urethra	84, 86
尿閉 urinary retention	86
尿路 urinary tract	87
尿瘻 urinary fistula	87
妊娠 pregnancy, gestation	94
妊娠悪阻 hyperemesis gravidarum	94
認知 cognition	97
認知機能 cognitive function	104, 106
認知症 dementia	97
認知の cognitive	97

ね

寝汗 night sweat	30
粘液 mucus	39, 51, 91
粘液性の mucous	39
粘着性の viscid	91
捻髪音 fine crackle	54
粘膜 mucosa, mucous membrane	26, 27, 29, 49, 51, 65, 72
粘膜疹 enanthema	29

の

脳 brain	18
嚢 sac	25
脳幹 brainstem	108
脳機能障害 brain dysfunction	97

膿細胞 pus cell	91
嚢腫 cyst	25
膿性の urulent	25
膿性物質 purulent matter	51
濃度 concentration	119
膿尿 pyuria	88
膿疱 pustule	25, 28
膿瘍 abscess	19

は

歯 tooth	68
パーキンソン病 Parkinson's disease	114
パーセンタイル percentile	17
胚 embryo	20
肺 lung	50, 51, 53
肺炎 pneumonia	56
肺胸膜 pulmonary pleura	55
背屈 dorsiflexion	112
排出物 discharge	45
排泄 excretion	85, 87
肺塞栓症 pulmonary embolism	56
肺組織 lung tissue	55
肺動脈 pulmonary artery	58, 60
排尿 urination	85, 86
排尿痛 dysuria	86
胚の embryonic	20
肺の pulmonary	55
胚発生 embryonic development	20
排便 bowel movement	76
排便する defecate	76
肺胞 alveoli (alveolus)	50, 54, 56
肺胞換気 alveolar ventilation	56
肺胞の alveolar	56
廃用 disuse	20
排卵 ovulation	92

日本語索引

白質　white matter … 113
白色瞳孔　leukocoria … 40
白帯下　leukorrhea … 91
白斑　leukoderma … 24
剥離　desquamation … 68
剥離した　desquamated … 68
暴露　exposure … 17, 39
破傷風　tetanus … 70
ばち指　clubbed fingers … 30
発音する　articulate … 110
発汗　perspiration, sweating … 30, 99
白血球　leukocyte, white blood cell … 68, 80, 81, 88
白血球減少　leukopenia … 81
白血球増加　leukocytosis … 81
白血病　leukemia … 81
発酵　fermentation … 77
発達障害　developmental disorder … 101
発熱　pyrexia, fever … 17
発話筋　speech muscle … 110
鼻　nose … 47
鼻ポリープ　nasal polyp … 49
パニック発作　panic attack … 99
バビンスキー徴候　Babinski sign … 112
腹　abdomen … 16
腫れ　swelling … 32, 54, 78, 119
斑　macule, patch … 23
半規管　semicircular canal … 44
半月弁　semilunar valve … 58, 61
瘢痕組織　scar tissue … 28
反射　reflex … 73
反射運動　reflex movement … 72
汎収縮期雑音　pansystolic murmur … 60
反跳圧痛　rebound tenderness … 73
半盲　hemianopia … 36

ビオー呼吸　Biot respiration … 53
皮下出血　subcutaneous hemorrhage … 23
皮下組織　subcutaneous tissue … 19, 22
皮下の　subcutaneous … 19
鼻腔　nasal cavity … 47, 50, 67, 48
皮溝　skin furrow … 22
鼻孔　nostril … 47, 50
尾骨　coccyx … 108
膝　knee … 16
皮脂　sebum … 31
肘　elbow … 16
脾腫　splenomegaly … 78
鼻出血　epistaxis, nosebleed … 49
脾臓　spleen … 67, 78
肥大　enlargement … 69, 74, 77, 78, 118, 119
泌尿器系　urinary system … 84
避妊　contraception … 93
鼻粘液　nasal mucus … 48
鼻粘膜　nasal mucous membrane … 48
皮膚　skin, cutis … 17, 18, 19, 23
皮膚緊張度　turgor … 19
皮膚疾患　cutaneous disorder … 30
皮膚の　cutaneous … 19
飛蚊症　muscae volitantes … 38
鼻閉　nasal obstruction … 48
非抱合型ビリルビン　unconjugated bilirubin … 87
肥満　obesity … 18
病因　etiology … 81
表在静脈　superficial vein … 65
病的な　morbid … 102
表皮　epidermis … 22, 27, 26
表皮細胞　epidermal cell … 27
表皮の　epidermal … 27

表皮剥離	excoriation		27
病変	lesion	23, 26, 33, 45, 109, 115	
びらん	erosion		26
鼻梁	nasal bridge		47, 48
ビリルビン	bilirubin		31, 87
ビリルビン尿	bilirubinuria		87
疲労	fatigue		38
鼻漏	rhinorrhea		48
貧血	anemia		81
頻呼吸	tachypnea		56
頻尿	urinary frequency		85
頻発月経	polymenorrhea		92
頻脈	tachycardia		62

ふ

不安	anxiety	99, 102
不快感	discomfort	18, 39
腹腔	abdominal cavity	32
複視	diplopia, double vision	38
副腎	adrenal gland	84
腹水	ascites	77
副鼻腔	paranasal sinus	47, 49
腹部	abdomen	73, 78
腹部腫瘤	abdominal mass	78
腹部膨満	abdominal distention	77
腹膜	peritoneum	77
腹膜腔	peritoneal cavity	77
腹膜の	peritoneal	77
腹鳴	borborygmus	77
ふくらはぎ	calf	64
浮腫	edema	19, 26, 42
不随意運動	involuntary movement	112
不随意の	involuntary	18
不正咬合	malocclusion	70
不正子宮出血	metrorrhagia	93

不整脈	arrhythmia	62
腹筋	abdominal muscle	73
舞踏運動	chorea	112
ブドウ糖	glucose	87, 119
不妊	infertility	93
不眠	insomnia	102
ブラウン・セカール症候群		
	Brown-Sequard syndrome	115
震え	shivering	17
ブルジンスキー徴候	Brudzinski sign	110
ブルンベルグ徴候	Blumberg sign	73
ブローカ失語	Broca's aphasia	103
分泌	secretion	31, 39, 48, 68, 75
分泌する	secrete	46
分泌物	secretion	54
噴門	cardia	75

へ

平滑筋	smooth muscle	53, 74
閉経	menopause	30
閉塞	obstruction	39, 72, 74, 88
壁細胞	parietal cell	75
ヘモグロビン	hemoglobin	81, 88
ヘルニア	hernia	91
ベル麻痺	Bell's palsy	109
便	stool	75, 76
変視症	metamorphopsia	38
変色	discoloration	31, 65
変色した	discolored	23
片側の	unilateral	109
便秘	constipation	76

ほ

防衛機制	defense mechanism	100
膀胱	bladder	84, 86, 87, 91, 95

日本語索引

抱合型ビリルビン　conjugated bilirubin ……… 87
芳香族の　aromatic ……… 70
膀胱瘤　cystocele ……… 91
房水フレア　aqueous flare ……… 39
房室ブロック　atrioventricular block … 64
房室弁　atrioventricular valve ……… 58, 59, 60, 61
膨疹　wheal ……… 26
膨張　distention ……… 72
乏尿　oliguria ……… 85
放屁　flatus ……… 71
飽和点　saturation point ……… 119
拇趾　great toe ……… 112
勃起不全　erectile dysfunction ……… 95
発疹　eruption, rash ……… 23, 29
母斑　nevus ……… 32
ホルネル症候群　Horner syndrome … 109
奔馬調律　gallop rhythm ……… 60

ま

膜　membrane ……… 25
膜性の　membranous ……… 25
摩擦音　friction sound ……… 55
末梢　periphery ……… 36
末梢気道　distal airway ……… 54
末梢神経障害　peripheral neuropathy … 115
末梢の　peripheral, distal ……… 36, 54
末端　extremity ……… 30
末端肥大症　acromegaly ……… 118
麻痺　paralysis ……… 109, 110
慢性の　chronic ……… 27

み

ミオクローヌス　myoclonus ……… 113

ミオグロビン　myoglobin ……… 88
ミオグロビン尿　myoglobinuria ……… 88
味覚　sense of taste ……… 68
味覚異常　dysgeusia ……… 68
耳　ear ……… 44
耳鳴り　tinnitus ……… 45
脈拍　pulse ……… 62, 63, 64
脈絡膜　choroid ……… 35

む

無為　abulia ……… 101
無意識　unconsciousness ……… 105
無害性雑音　innocent murmur ……… 60
無顆粒白血球　agranulocyte ……… 80
無汗症　anhidrosis ……… 109
無月経　amenorrhea ……… 92
無呼吸　apnea ……… 52, 53, 56
無胆汁便　acholic stool ……… 76
無動　akinesia ……… 104
無動の　akinetic ……… 104
無動無言症　akinetic mutism ……… 104
無尿　anuria ……… 85
胸　chest ……… 16
胸やけ　pyrosis, heartburn ……… 71, 74

め

眼　eye, oculus ……… 35, 38
メズサの頭　caput medusae ……… 73
眼の　ocular ……… 38
めまい　vertigo ……… 19
めまい感　dizziness ……… 115
免疫　immunity ……… 17
免疫系　immune system ……… 17
免疫疾患　immune disorder ……… 78
免疫の　immune ……… 17

も

毛細血管	capillary	23, 27, 31
毛細血管拡張	telangiectasia	27
妄想	delusion	98, 106
盲腸	cecum	67
毛乳頭	hair papilla	22
盲斑部	blind spot	35
毛包	hair follicle	22, 28
毛母基	hair matrix	22
網膜	retina	35, 36, 40
毛様体	ciliary body	35
毛様体小帯	ciliary zonule	35

や

夜間頻尿	nocturia	85
山羊声	egophony	55
薬物	drug	30, 33
やせ	emaciation	18
夜尿症	nocturnal enuresis	86
夜盲症	nyctalopia, night blindness	37

ゆ

有機酸	organic acid	69
幽門	pylorus	74, 75
幽門の	pyloric	74
幽門部	pyloric area	75
幽門弁	pyloric valve	74

よ

葉気管支	lobar bronchi	50
溶血	hemolysis	88
腰神経	lumbar nerve	108
ヨウ素欠乏症	iodine deficiency	119
腰椎	lumbar vertebrae	108
腰部の	lumbar	116

ら

落屑	desquamation	27
卵管	uterine tube	90
卵巣	ovary	90, 92

り

離人症	depersonalization	100
立毛筋	arrector pili muscle	22
リポ蛋白	lipoprotein	119
隆起	elevation	24, 25, 26
流産	abortion	94
流涙症	epiphora	39
両価性	ambivalence	100
良性の	benign	24
両側麻痺	diplegia	105
臨床徴候	clinical sign	110
鱗屑	scale, squama	27
リンパ管	lymphatic vessel	88
リンパ球	lymphocyte	80
リンパ節	lymph node	32
リンパ節腫脹	lymphadenopathy	32

る・れ

涙道	lacrimal passage	39
類白血病反応	leukemoid reaction	81
連続性雑音	continuous murmur	61

ろ・わ

漏出液	transudate	52
肋骨	costa	55
肋骨胸膜	costal pleura	55
肋骨の	costal	55
ロンベルク徴候	Romberg sign	114
彎曲	curvature	116

Profile

著者

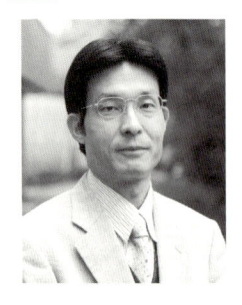

近藤 真治（こんどう しんじ）
愛知医科大学看護学部教授（医療英語）

1965年米国カリフォルニア州生まれ．上智大学外国語学部英語学科卒業．ミシガン州立大学大学院コミュニケーション研究科修士課程修了．岐阜経済大学経済学部専任講師，福井大学医学部助教授，同教授を経て，現在は愛知医科大学看護学部教授（医療英語）．主な著書（共著）に，『コミュニケーション不安の形成と治療』（ナカニシヤ出版），『からだの英語集中マスター』（メジカルビュー社）など．

英文校閲・ナレーター

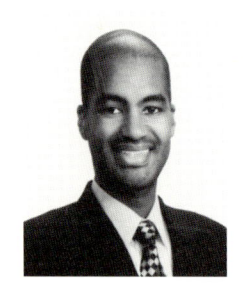

Wayne Malcolm
福井大学語学センター 講師

Wayne Malcolm is a senior assistant professor at University of Fukui where he works in the Language Center providing English language instruction and conducting research in various areas. His primary research efforts focus on listening and speaking skills, judgemental and nonjudgemental attitudes in the classroom, as well as study abroad in higher education curriculum. Originally from Cornwall, New York in the United States he has been living in Japan since September 2002. Married in 2007 he and his wife have one daughter.

編集協力

飯野 哲（いいの さとし）
福井大学医学部教授
（形態機能医科学講座人体解剖学・神経科学領域）

1966年山梨県生まれ．山梨医科大学医学科卒業．名古屋大学医学部助手，福井大学医学部助教授を経て，福井大学医学部教授（人体解剖学・神経科学領域）．解剖学組織学を専門とし，消化管の組織学的研究に携わる．

その症候、英語で言えますか？
はじめに覚える335症候とついでに覚える1000の関連語

2014年11月15日 第1刷発行	著 者	近藤真治
	英文校閲・ナレーター	Wayne Malcolm
	編集協力	飯野 哲
	発行人	一戸裕子
	発行所	株式会社 羊 土 社
		〒101-0052 東京都千代田区神田小川町2-5-1 TEL 03 (5282) 1211 FAX 03 (5282) 1212 E-mail eigyo@yodosha.co.jp URL http://www.yodosha.co.jp/
Ⓒ YODOSHA CO., LTD. 2014 Printed in Japan	装幀・本文デザイン	株式会社サンビジネス
	イラスト	小山琴美（株式会社ツグミ）
ISBN978-4-7581-1760-9	印刷所	日経印刷株式会社

本書に掲載する著作物の複製権，上映権，譲渡権，公衆送信権（送信可能化権を含む）は（株）羊土社が保有します．
本書を無断で複製する行為（コピー，スキャン，デジタルデータ化など）は，著作権法上での限られた例外（「私的使用のための複製」など）を除き禁じられています．研究活動，診療を含み業務上使用する目的で上記の行為を行うことは大学，病院，企業などにおける内部的な利用であっても，私的使用には該当せず，違法です．また私的使用のためであっても，代行業者等の第三者に依頼して上記の行為を行うことは違法となります．

JCOPY ＜（社）出版者著作権管理機構 委託出版物＞
本書の無断複写は著作権法上での例外を除き禁じられています．複写される場合は，そのつど事前に，（社）出版者著作権管理機構（TEL 03-3513-6969，FAX 03-3513-6979，e-mail：info@jcopy.or.jp）の許諾を得てください．

羊土社のオススメ書籍

Dr.リトルが教える
医学英語スピーキングが素晴らしく上達する方法

症例プレゼンや日常臨床,学会発表などで聞き手を惹きつける話し方の秘訣と英文例

ドーリックリトル／著,
町　淳二／監訳

アメリカ臨床留学を成功させた日本人医師はみんな,リトル先生に学んでいた！野口アラムナイ（野口医学研究所同窓生）による翻訳で,英語による症例プレゼンが絶対上手くなる秘訣を教えます.さあ,今すぐ誌上留学！

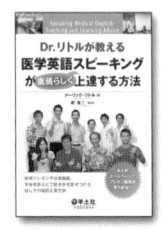

- 定価（本体3,400円＋税）　A5判
- 180頁　ISBN 978-4-7581-1728-9

やさしい英語で外来診療

聞きもらしのない問診のコツ

大山　優／監,
安藤克利／著,
Jason F. Hardy, 遠藤玲／協力・ナレーター

英会話は苦手…という方にオススメ！外来の流れに沿って,シンプルでも患者さんにしっかり伝わる口語表現を解説.症状ごとに必要な情報を確実に聞き取るコツがよくわかる！日常ですぐ活かせる一冊です.音声CDつき.

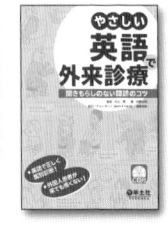

- 定価（本体3,400円＋税）　A5判
- 246頁　ISBN 978-4-7581-1726-5

臨床につながる
解剖学イラストレイテッド

松村讓兒／著,
土屋一洋／協力

疾患のなりたちや治療法から,人体の構造と役割を楽しく学べる教科書.イメージしやすいイラストと豊富な臨床画像,親しみやすい文章で臨床でも役立つ解剖学知識が自然と身に付く！解剖のおさらいにもオススメ.

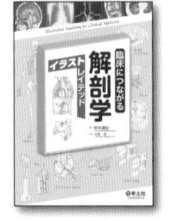

- 定価（本体6,200円＋税）　B5判
- 348頁　ISBN 978-4-7581-2025-8

研究者のための
思考法 10のヒント

知的しなやかさで
人生の壁を乗り越える

島岡　要／著

天職を探している,創造的な研究者になりたい…誰もが抱える悩みが突破口に変わる！「研究者の仕事術」でおなじみの著者が,社会学・心理学など複眼的視点から導いた"よく生きる"ためのポイントをわかりやすく解説.

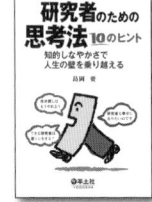

- 定価（本体2,700円＋税）　A5判
- 222頁　ISBN 978-4-7581-2037-1

発行　羊土社　YODOSHA
〒101-0052　東京都千代田区神田小川町2-5-1　TEL 03(5282)1211　FAX 03(5282)1212
E-mail：eigyo@yodosha.co.jp
URL：http://www.yodosha.co.jp/

ご注文は最寄りの書店,または小社営業部まで